DR MEGAN ROSSI

Eat Yourself Healthy

An easy-to-digest guide to health and happiness from the inside out

PHOTOGRAPHY BY EMMA CROMAN

PENGUIN LIFE
an imprint of
PENGUIN BOOKS

PENGUIN LIFE

UK | USA | Canada | Ireland | Australia

India | New Zealand | South Africa

Penguin Life is part of the Penguin Random House group of companies whose addresses can be found at global.penguinrandomhouse.com.

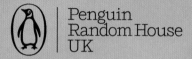

First published 2019
001

Text copyright © Megan Rossi, 2019
Photography © Emma Croman, 2019
Design and art direction by nic&lou

Colour repro by ALTAimage Ltd
Printed in Italy by Printer Trento S.r.l.

A CIP catalogue record for this book is available from the British Library

ISBN: 978–0–241–35508–4

www.greenpenguin.co.uk

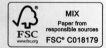

Penguin Random House is committed to a sustainable future for our business, our readers and our planet. This book is made from Forest Stewardship Council® certified paper.

Eat
Yourself
Healthy

740007439842

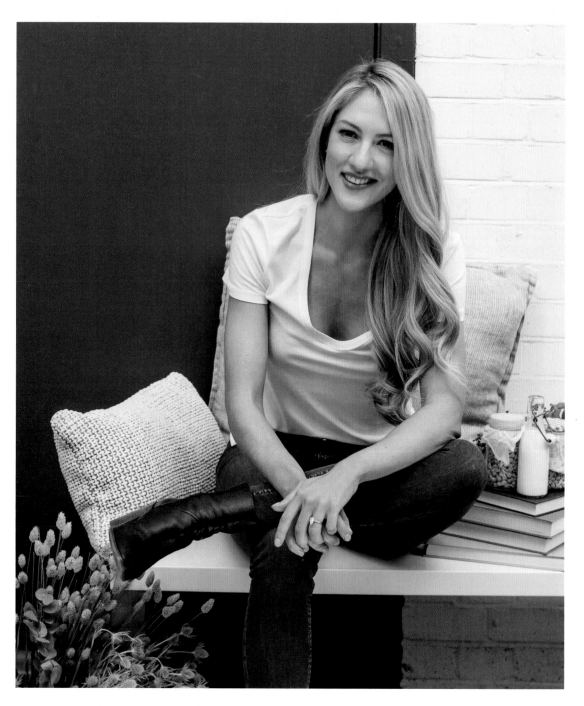

In loving memory of my sister Justine, nephew Boyd, and grandma Ruth
– you inspire me every day. This book is for you.

Contents

INTRODUCTION: THE START OF SOMETHING BEAUTIFUL   **6**

/ 1.   UNDERSTANDING YOUR GUT   **12**

/ 2.   YOUR INNER UNIVERSE OF MICROBES   **22**

/ 3.   NUTRITION FOR THE GUT   **38**

/ 4.   COMMON COMPLAINTS   **78**

/ 5.   FOOD INTOLERANCES   **108**

/ 6.   IRRITABLE BOWEL SYNDROME   **136**

/ 7.   BEYOND DIET   **158**

/ 8.   IN THE KITCHEN   **186**

CONCLUSION: YOUR GUT HEALTH ACTION PLAN   **282**

Indexes   **292**

With Thanks   **304**

Introduction

The start of something beautiful . . .

THE GUT. A simple yet powerful three-letter word and something I have come to think of as beautiful. Yes, I know what you're thinking, it's where poop comes from, for crying out loud! I get it, I used to think the same, but by the time you get to the end of this book, I'm going to have you talking about your gut with a new-found level of admiration and even a dash of excitement. So, let me introduce you . . .

Say hello to what we nerdy scientists call your gut microbiota (GM). I'm aware it's not the sexiest of terms – let's go with GM moving forward. This wonderful, complex and thriving community is made up of the trillions of microbes that call your intestine home. Your GM is incredibly powerful – in fact, this newly appreciated organ is pretty much essential to whatever your health goal is. It's not only capable of thousands of functions, going well beyond what we could achieve on our own, but it has also been linked with successful weight management, improved fitness levels, healthier skin, boosted immunity and even our happiness.

What really blows my mind is that, unlike our genetic make-up, over which we have no control, we have the ability to shape our GM simply by how we treat it – which means that a big part of our personal health is in our hands. However, as with all landmark scientific discoveries, there are those who will seek to take advantage of people looking for help by twisting the truth and promoting over-hyped, sham, gut-boosting products. But don't let this detract from the fact that the field of gut health is based on real science and has the potential to have a measurable impact on your health and happiness. In this book I want to create a safe place to learn about the gut that's all about keeping it real by sticking with the evidence.

The concept of gut health is really nothing new. You see, our GM is just one part of overall gut health. Other major aspects include its role in our immunity (70 per cent of immune cells live along the gut), as well as in digestion and the absorption of nutrients, which, if not working right, can lead to an array of nutrition deficiencies and negative health consequences. So, clearly, taking the time to understand and look after our gut is one of the best ways we can invest in our future.

There is a growing and frankly concerning trend towards generic, over-simplified, one-size-fits-all gut health recommendations. I'm sure you've all heard it before: 'Eat more probiotics',

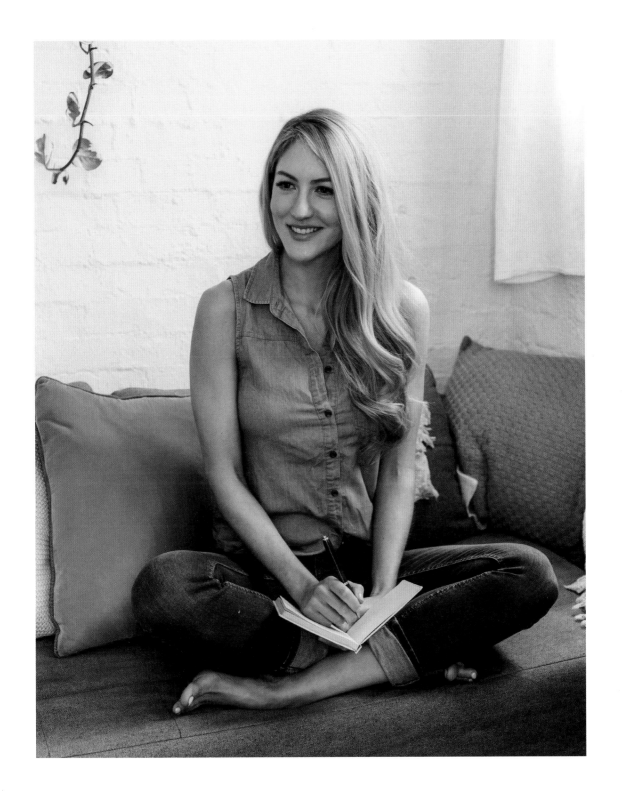

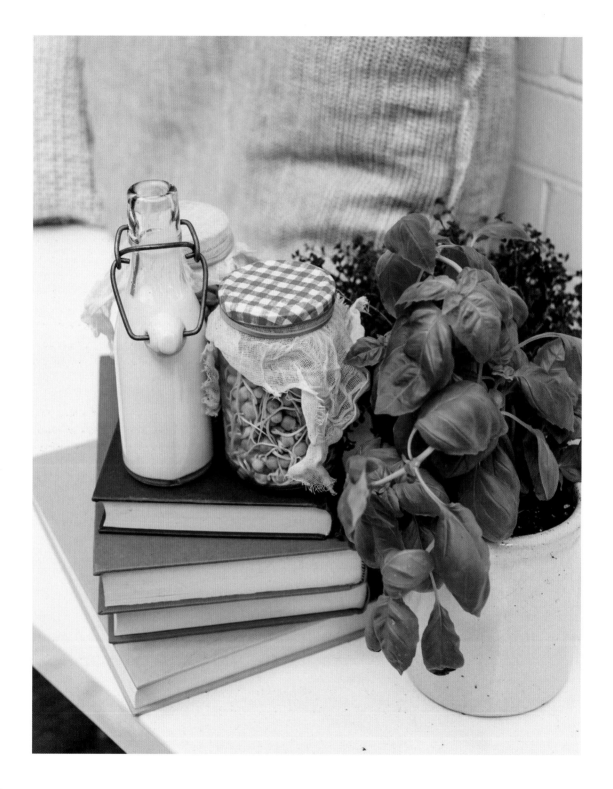

'Eat more fermented foods' . . . and on and on. These messages, although I'm sure they're mostly given with only good intentions, can actually do more harm than good. An example of this is the contradictory message that everyone should be eating more prebiotics if they want good gut health. My research, and research done by others, has clearly demonstrated that adding extra prebiotics into your diet can in fact trigger gut symptoms in around 15–20 per cent of the population, particularly those with irritable bowel syndrome (IBS). Yes, of course increasing prebiotics in your diet can be good for you, but it really does depend on where you are on your gut-health journey.

How do you know what's right for you? In this book, we'll go through several assessments (just as I would in my clinic) to help you determine where your gut health is currently at and then, based on this, we'll explore a range of tools and strategies so that you can formulate your own evidence-based gut health action plan. All assessments in this book can be found on my website, www.TheGutHealthDoctor.com, and your scores recorded in your gut-health action plan on page 283.

I do need to prepare you, though: things are going to get real personal – there's no hiding behind a generic meal plan here. This book is written in a way that I hope not only makes you fall in love with your gut (as I have with mine), but also helps you get the most out of it, whether it's managing existing gut symptoms or maximizing your gut health's impact on other organs, such as your brain. Let's face it, it's the same as most relationships: if you don't give it enough love and attention, things can turn pretty ugly.

My goal in writing this book is to give you a reference guide to your gut – how it works, how to look after it, how to maximize its potential and, importantly, how to manage it with simple steps when it's not functioning quite right. Using the right balance of science, anecdotes, practical strategies and tasty recipes, I will take you on a journey of discovery, leaving you with tangible take-home messages and a step-by-step action plan that will make a meaningful and measurable difference to your everyday life. The book will also equip you with the skills needed to separate the facts from the fiction without getting too 'sciencey' on you – promise.

It's time to get excited: your journey of self-discovery and gut love is about to begin!

Assessment: 'IS MY GUT HEALTHY?'

This has to be the most common question I get asked, and it's one I never give a simple 'yes' or 'no' answer to. There's no single measure we can use to assess our gut health. However, with the right set of tools, you can get a pretty good idea of how healthy your gut is without having to step a foot outside your door. Head to www.TheGutHealthDoctor.com to complete your first assessment, then check back with this book.

My Story

I grew up on a farm just outside of Cairns, Australia, where our lifestyle was inherently supportive of good gut health – we played in the dirt and lived on fresh, home-grown produce – yet my first conscious memory of the gut wasn't a happy one. It was during my nutrition and dietetics undergraduate degree, when my grandma, the most caring soul, was diagnosed with bowel cancer. I remember watching on helplessly as she bravely battled through chemo and surgery – I hated the gut for doing this to her. Grandma fought on as long as she could but lost her battle in 2009, during my final year of university. I still vividly recall sitting in a lecture at university soon after she'd passed, being taught about the early warning signs of bowel cancer and thinking to myself, I wonder, if talking about our bowels wasn't such a socially taboo topic, would my granny have spoken up earlier and still be here today? The statistics suggested yes, she would be.

A few years later, those negative emotions surrounding the gut resurfaced. I was working in a hospital as a dietitian and was struck by the sheer number of patients with kidney disease who were complaining of gut issues. I really struggled to get my head around how, whereas my grandma had her disease in her actual gut, all these patients with their various kidney diseases also suffered with such prominent gut issues. I searched just about every textbook and research paper I could find and still couldn't give my patients a proper answer. I couldn't let it rest. I was determined to get to the bottom of it and, before I knew it, I found myself signing away my early twenties to answer this very question – was there a link between the kidneys and the gut? Fast-forward three years, and it turns out there is! It's something we now call the gut–kidney axis. But my fascination with the subject didn't stop there. I was fortunate to also work with Olympic athletes and a number of company CEOs, and they got me thinking

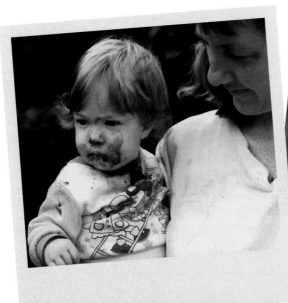

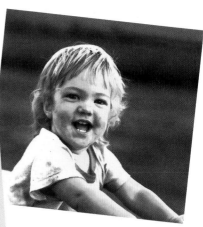

about the link between the gut and the brain (commonly referred to as the gut–brain axis). I noticed that those who were suffering the greatest levels of stress were the ones suffering the most significant gut issues. It also became clear that, by nourishing the gut and caring for it, people could improve their lives in very real and often surprising ways, and I could help them to do this. This was the turning point in my relationship with the gut – my eyes were finally opened to its power and promise.

So why this book? I went into research to make a difference, but a year into my post-doctoral post I became frustrated that, despite the incredible research that was being done, it was the unfounded and potentially dangerous fad nutritional messages that were being almost force-fed to the public. I was seeing extremes in my clinic, with some people essentially starving themselves because they'd had (invalid) food-intolerance tests and were scared to eat anything, while others (and I'm talking really intelligent people) were overdosing on herbal supplements in order to 'boost' their gut health because they'd read about the gut–brain axis and wanted that extra 'edge' at work. Right before my eyes, I was seeing that the very thing I had come to admire – the gut – was being misrepresented and so destroying people's health. It was this injustice that ignited my passion for science communication. This, along with your endless support on social media, continues to drive my mission to help people find inspiration and take the evidence-based steps to a happy, healthy life. But that's quite enough about my story. This book is all about your journey.

So, let's get started!

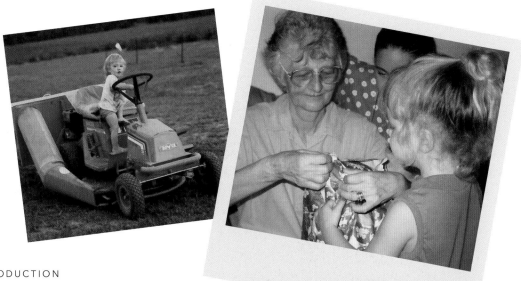

CHAPTER 1

Understanding your gut

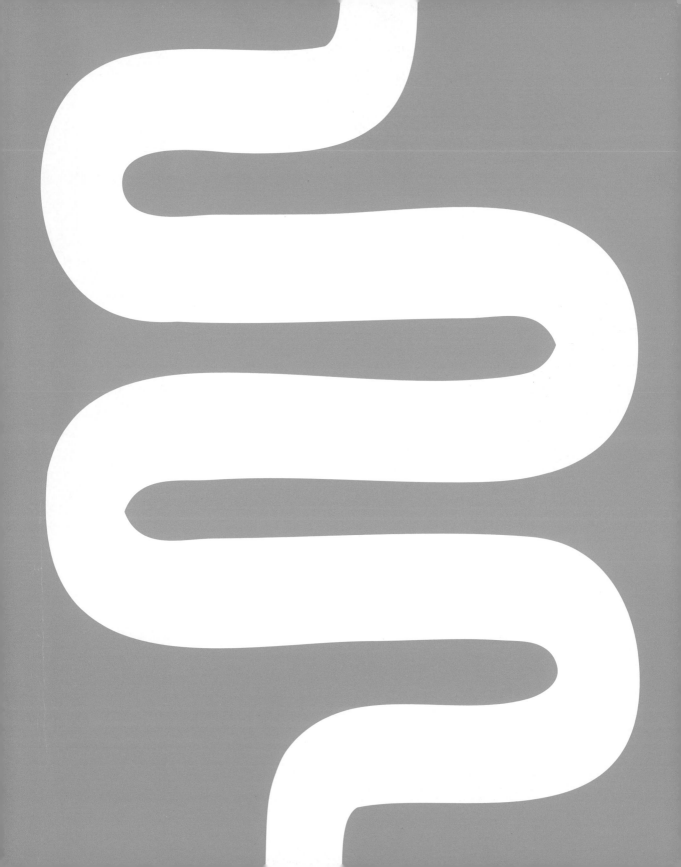

Understanding your gut

One of the most important and fundamental things you will ever learn about nutrition is this – what actually happens to food once it enters your mouth.

Why is this knowledge so important? For those who suffer with gut issues, it can help you understand the possible causes. This not only helps you become a better detective when we come to try and identify your triggers in Chapter 5, but also, having this improved awareness of what goes on inside us can offer a huge amount of relief. Gut issues aside, by understanding how your body handles food, you're also safeguarding yourself against the many nutrition myths out there, for instance, that sucrose (aka sugar) is bad for your gut microbes. (Spoiler alert: it's absorbed higher up your intestine, so it doesn't reach the majority of them.)

Despite the hype around our gut microbiota (GM), gut health relates to our entire digestive tract. Which means gut health is not just about the microbes but also governs the digestion of food and absorption of nutrients and maintains most of our immune system. In fact, only a small section of our nine-metre-long factory line (aka our digestive tract) contains the bulk of our GM.

Our digestive tract is the barrier between our body and the environment, which means that food doesn't really get into our body until long after we've eaten it and it has passed through our gut lining's defence barrier and into our bloodstream. If you think about it, this is a huge responsibility for our gut, and it explains why it's equipped with an incredible 70 per cent of our body's immune cells.

So, let's take a look at what happens to food as it travels through our body . . .

In your mouth . . .

This is where digestion begins. Food is not only physically broken down in our mouth into smaller bits by our teeth; it is also chemically broken down, thanks to special proteins in our saliva known as enzymes. For example, if you keep a piece of white bread in your mouth for long enough, the enzymes start to break down the complex carbohydrates (starch) and release simple carbohydrates (sugars). As this chemical process happens in your mouth, you will notice that the bread will start to taste sweet – give it a try.

In your oesophagus . . .

Once you swallow your chewed food, it slides down your food pipe (aka oesophagus). To stop the food going down your windpipe, which is right next door to the food pipe, when we swallow a special trapdoor known as the epiglottis slams shut over our windpipe. Have you ever tried to speak and swallow at the same time? It's impossible, without choking, and that's all thanks to our epiglottis.

In your stomach . . .

As food travels down your food pipe, before it gets into the stomach it needs to pass another delightfully designed circular ring of muscle that acts as a gateway known as the lower oesophageal sphincter. As food moves into each of the next three sections of your digestive tract, it passes through another gateway, or sphincter, at each stage. These sphincters are important, as they keep the different sections separate from each other. Sometimes, however, they don't shut or open properly, which can result in common complaints such as acid reflux and other conditions which we will discuss in Chapter 4.

You can think of the stomach as a kind of washing machine, because it not only physically churns and throws food around like a washing machine does our clothes, but it also releases detergent-like chemicals. They include:

1. ENZYMES: to break up our food

2. ACID: to kill off microbes trying to invade our body

3. HORMONES: which not only trigger the gut muscles to get their act together and start contracting but also let us know when we are full or hungry

It's in your stomach that your once-solid meal will be transformed to have a more smoothie-like consistency (known as chyme). Once formed, this smoothie mix makes its way from the stomach into the next section of our digestive tract: the small intestine.

In your small intestine . . .

'Small intestine' is bit of a funny name for it because it's the longest part of our digestive tract, reaching close to seven metres in length when stretched out. If it was laid out flat, it would cover the surface area of nearly half a badminton court! How it achieves this impressive surface area is down to the tiny, carpet-like projections (villi and microvilli) which exist along our small intestine. These projections are vital for nutrient absorption, that is, the movement of nutrients from our gut into our circulation. In scenarios where these finger-like projections are flattened or squashed, such as in undiagnosed coeliac disease, you are likely to suffer from nutrient deficiencies, partly because your small intestine just doesn't have the surface area that is needed to absorb all the nutrients from your food. Before the smoothie mix can move into our circulation it needs to be broken down further, which is where the pancreas comes in. Our pancreas is another organ that feeds into our small intestine, and acts like a busy factory producing enzymes that help digest our food as well as hormones which help control how much sugar is in your blood.

To further assist with digestion, yet another detergent-like mix, known as bile acids, is made by our liver, and stored in a small pouch known as the gallbladder. Bile is secreted into our small intestine and helps with fat digestion and absorption.

In addition to the enzymes released by our pancreas, the lining of our small intestine also contains enzymes that break down food. For example, lactase, an enzyme that breaks down lactose (a type of sugar found in milk from animals), perches on the lining of your small intestine, waiting to do its job at a moment's notice.

After around two to six hours in your small intestine – depending what and how much you've eaten, as well as how your gut muscles are working – the unabsorbed bits (including my own personal favourite nutrient, dietary fibre) will move through the next gateway (this one is called the ileocaecal valve) and on into the large intestine. As the food passes through this gateway, our large intestine acts a bit like a watchdog and keeps an eye on the sort of things that are passing through. If it starts to notice under-digested food coming through, it pulls the brake on our upper-gut movements. This system is known as the ileal brake and is an important feedback system that helps maximize nutrient absorption in the small intestine. One of the side effects of this is decreased appetite, which explains why often, when we have diarrhoea, we also lose our appetite.

In your large intestine . . .

THE LARGE INTESTINE IS RESPONSIBLE FOR FOUR MAIN THINGS:

1. HYDRATION: Your large intestine reabsorbs fluid and electrolytes. During this process your gut contents turn from liquid to solid and the longer your poop-to-be is in the large intestine, the more water it absorbs and therefore the more solid the poop.

2. OUR GM RESIDENTS: Your large intestine houses the trillions of microbes that make up our GM. Although we have microbes scattered throughout our digestive tract, this is where the main bulk of microbes hang out. We'll chat more about this in Chapter 2.

3. NUTRIENT ABSORPTION: You know how I said that most of the nutrient absorption occurs in the small intestine? Well, that is indeed true, but the large intestine also plays a pivotal role. This is because our GM rather handily helps digest things that are indigestible to human enzymes, such as fibre. In doing so, our microbes produce messenger molecules that are capable of many things, such as messaging our brain to say, 'Okay, you can stop eating now, thanks, we're full,' as well as reducing gut inflammation, and much more.

4. WASTE COMPACTOR: The end of our large intestine – the rectum – stores and compacts the waste produced by the body, including the parts of dead red blood cells which make our poop brown. Once our brain sends a message to give our rectum the all-clear, the accumulated waste is released through our final digestive-tract gateway and out through the muscular opening known as the anus.

Unlike our small intestine, our large intestine plays the slow and steady game. This is why undigested foods take around twelve to thirty hours to move through it, despite the large intestine being around four times shorter than the small intestine.

How the gut moves

We've discussed a lot about what happens in each part of the gut, but we haven't yet addressed how food is actually moved through it.

Your first thought might be that it is all down to gravity, but remember, the gut is close to nine metres of folded intestines, which means that sometimes food has to move against gravity. To allow for this, our digestive tract is coated with both long and circular muscles which contract in a symphony of orchestrated patterns to guide food on its extraordinary journey through the gut. This is known as motility.

Several 'programmed' movements are responsible for the transport of food between different parts of the digestive tract, and they differ depending on whether we have eaten or not. One of the two basic types of programmed movements is peristaltic waves, which pump food along the gut; the other is segmentation contractions, which help to mix all the gut contents together, including food and enzymes, like a big pot of warm soup.

Programmed movements may be coordinated into higher-level motility patterns. The best example is the migrating motor complex (MMC), which typically moves from the stomach through the small intestine, essentially sweeping the intestine clean between meals. The MMC is like those trucks that come out to clear up after a major road race or event. It sweeps any leftover bits of rubbish into the large intestine, as well as any microbes that may have crept up unannounced from our large intestine. Next time you hear your belly rumble, don't stress out, it's likely just your intestinal 'housekeeper', aka the MMC, doing its thing. This movement occurs every forty-five minutes to two hours, but only between meals, that is, in the fasted state, and generally when you are sleeping. It's one of the many reasons why sleeping is so important for the gut; we'll touch on this in Chapter 7. Dysfunction of the MMC may also play a role in some types of gut issue, such as small intestinal bacterial overgrowth (SIBO), which we'll discuss on page 156.

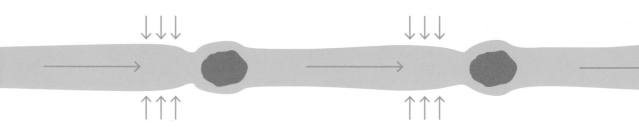

Mass movement is another type of programmed movement and occurs between six and ten times a day in the large intestine. This is the final 'kick', so to speak, propelling your formed poop into your rectum, ready for evacuation. One of the main triggers of this mass movement is eating (known as the gastro-colic reflex, that urge to go you often feel after eating). It's also worth noting that different foods are thought to have different effects on this type of movement; for instance, fat and carbohydrate are more likely to stimulate the movement than protein. Gentle exercise, such as going for a walk, particularly after a meal, is also known to activate this type of movement. Mass movements are put on hold overnight but pick up again sharply in the morning, which also explains why many people poop in the morning.

SO. . . what makes your gut muscles contract?

Our gut is really pretty impressive in that, unlike any other organ, it can function independently of our brain. This means that our gut can go about its business, digesting and moving food along, without our brain telling it to do so. This high-level function is all thanks to our gut's impressive network of hundreds of millions of nerves, known as the enteric nervous system. This explains why our gut has been dubbed our second brain.

Despite this impressive level of independence, a two-way communication normally occurs between the enteric nervous system and our primary ('big') brain. Much of this communication occurs via our parasympathetic nerves, which is often referred to as the 'rest and digest' response, and our sympathetic nerves, which take over when in 'fight or flight' response. Typically, when our body feels stressed (because our brain is telling it that we are), the parasympathetic nervous system is regulated downwards and so gut function is reduced, because all the blood rushes to our muscles to get them ready to fight (or flee). When we are relaxed, blood goes back into our gut to support digestion. This may explain why some people struggle to poop when they're stressed. Of course, that's not always the case: for some stress can trigger diarrhoea, and this is because of overactive or hyper-responsive gut-motility programming, as well as secretion of additional fluid into the gut – the gut–brain link is clearly complex!

Defence system

The gut is the reason we're not all bedridden and defeated by infection every time we eat or step outside. Like all powerhouses, our body has two main lines of defence, the front-line defence being our intestinal wall, which acts as a physical barrier to foreign invaders (like a bouncer at the door outside a club), and the second-line defence being the more sophisticated and dynamic immune system (think security cameras, alarms and so on).

The wall of our intestine is made up of a barrier of cells (think of a row of doors) that are effectively secured by tight junctions (club bouncers). Our intestinal wall serves a dual purpose; like the door and the bouncer who guards it, this allows the passage of the good guys (nutrients) and keeps out the bad guys (pathogens). These tight junctions can become weak, or loose, allowing unwanted nasties to sneak across the intestinal wall. Scientists call this intestinal hyperpermeability; a more user-friendly term is 'leaky gut'. Thankfully, even if a pathogen does make it through the first line, our immune system is primed and waiting to pounce, triggering a cascade of events both within and outside our gut to shut down any nasty invasions.

Your immune system is amazingly complex, involving a high-level network of cells, tissues and organs that work together to fight off invaders. The 70 per cent of immune tissue that lies within our gut – our gut-associated lymphoid tissue (GALT) – has a particularly important job, because our digestive tract is the most popular gateway into the body. It's a pretty tough job, really: the team is constantly on patrol, sifting through millions of foreign cells each day (from things we eat and drink, as well as our resident GM), discriminating between harmless (e.g. proteins in foods and friendly microbes) and potentially dangerous ones (e.g. toxins and pathogenic microbes).

The GALT isn't just important for fighting invaders, it also keeps the rest of our cells and GM in check. This includes performance-assessing old cells that have been subject to extensive wear and tear (and deciding which ones should be made to retire), and good microbes which 'act up' and find themselves in the wrong place, that is, crossing the gut barrier.

What happens when things go wrong, when this delicate balance between fighting off the bad guys (immunity) and recognizing the good guys (immune tolerance) is compromised? If the balance tends more towards immunity, conditions such as food allergies (innocent food proteins are mistakenly tagged as a threat) and auto-immune diseases (where it's the body's own tissue that gets tagged) arise. If it tends more towards immune tolerance (often referred to as immune-compromised), as in the case of during certain cancer treatments, e.g. chemotherapy, your body can be more vulnerable to invasion by the bad guys, which may lead to severe infections.

What about your GM? They have a major role in our body's defence system; in fact, without them, our immune system would, frankly, be pretty weak. This is because the microbes train our immune system from birth. This explains the 'hygiene hypothesis', which states that being too clean, particularly in infancy, means that you are exposed to fewer microbes, and so your GM diversity (the number of different types of microbes you house) decreases. As a result, the diversity of the 'coaching' of your immune system is also reduced. This is one explanation for why rates of allergy and auto-immune conditions are reaching epidemic levels in the Western world.

Assessment: LISTENING TO YOUR GUT FEELINGS

Have you ever sat down and had a two-way conversation with your gut? You may be surprised by how much you learn from simply taking the time to listen to your gut.

Although most of us have a sense of when our gut is not functioning quite right, we rarely pinpoint details of the specific symptoms. Doing so can provide invaluable insight and is really worth taking time over. It can not only help you troubleshoot in a more systematic (and therefore helpful) way, but if you do end up needing to see your GP or dietitian, it's a great source of information that you can provide, allowing them more time to carry out a thorough assessment in the short time they have to see you. At the start of all my consultations I get my patients to fill out this questionnaire to help focus our intervention on the areas most important to them.

Head to www.TheGutHealthDoctor.com to complete the 'Listening to Your Gut Feelings' assessment and 'Checking in with Your Poop' assessments. Remember to record your results in your gut health action plan on page 283.

CHAPTER 2

Your inner universe of microbes

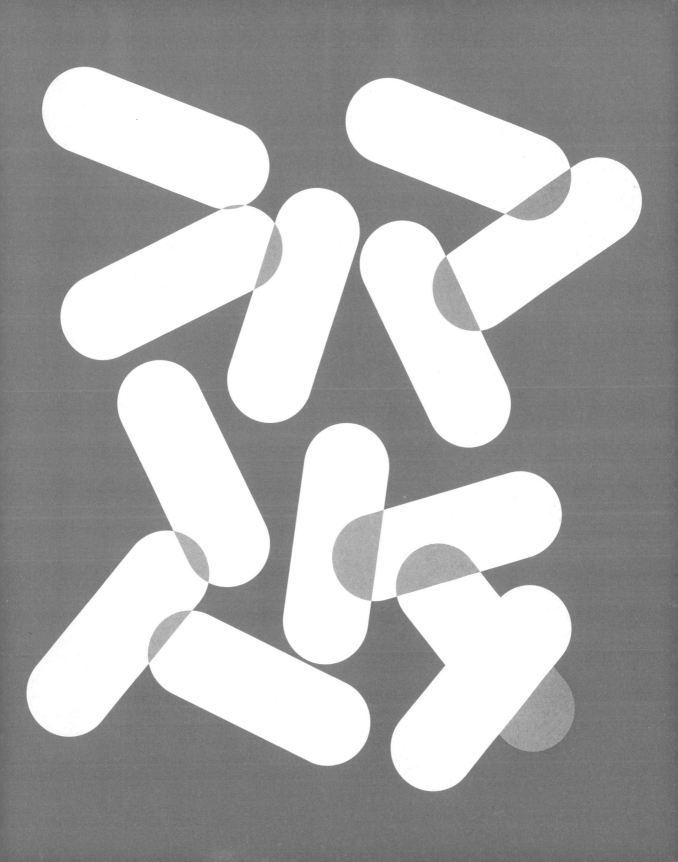

Your inner universe of microbes

Microbes have been around for billions of years, humans less than a million. They can multiply in minutes, survive and thrive in every habitat on earth, from volcanic explosions to glaciers; they've killed more people than all wars and human accidents combined (not a stat to be proud of, but relevant, nonetheless). Perhaps most humbling of all, without microbes, we couldn't survive – but, without humans, microbes would do just fine.

Admittedly, this does paint our relationship as a little one-sided, but I can promise you, deep down, your microbes want to see you thrive. As long as you show them some love and appreciation, like all close friends, they will have your back.

When I talk about microbes I'm not just talking about our gut microbiota (GM), which we will cover in detail shortly. Our body is in fact like a mini-ecosystem of different microbial communities. They live in us – in our lungs, our nose, our urinary tract, and so on – and they also live on us, like a second skin. To microbes, our armpits are like a tropical forest, our backs like a wide open field, and distinct communities populate each area.

Skin microbiota

We each have billions of microbes living on our skin. We also emit our own distinct cloud of microbes wherever we go, and this is unique, like a fingerprint. This microbial fingerprint, which can't be hidden from others simply by wearing gloves, has grabbed the attention of criminologists as an exciting new forensic tool to hunt down criminals. Perhaps not surprisingly, our skin microbiota also plays a role in common skin conditions like acne, eczema and certain skin cancers. But before we go getting our hopes up, the ways in which we can manipulate our skin microbes to help prevent and manage those skin conditions are still poorly understood. In terms of preventing eczema in infants, there is supportive evidence that taking probiotics during pregnancy may reduce your baby's risk by up to 50 per cent; however, for treating eczema and acne, studies that have been carried out to date indicate that probiotics don't seem to help. Instead, what is more promising is topical probiotics, where the bacteria are directly placed on the skin. But it's still only early days, so I'd be a little sceptical for now if you come across companies selling 'probiotic' skincare. Regarding skin cancers, recent studies in mice have suggested that a specific species of bacteria (*Staphylococcus epidermidis*) was able to produce a chemical that protected the mice against developing skin cancer. Although this finding has yet to be replicated in humans, it suggests that a specific skin microbiota may indeed play an important role in protecting against skin cancer. I am hopeful that in the near future there will be evidence-based products targeting the skin microbiota. But in the meantime, it's best to safeguard yourself by asking about the human research that has been done (not test-tube or animal studies) before handing over your hard-earned cash.

Oral microbiota

There is also a community of microbes which claim residence in our mouth. Although notorious for causing bad breath and dental issues, rest assured that this is the doing of only a select few troublemakers; the vast majority of microbes work to support a healthy mouth environment. They not only act as the bodyguard to our GM, they also play several other roles in maintaining our general health. This includes metabolizing specific nutrients such as nitrates from plants like beetroot, which can help manage high blood pressure and support heart health.

So how do we look after these guys? Standard oral hygiene like brushing our teeth properly and regularly and not overdoing it on added sugars – think fizzy drinks and sweets – is a good place to start. One study did report that with each 'intimate' kiss we transfer an average of 80 million bacteria. This suggests that perhaps our partner's diet could also have an impact on our own microbes. I do vividly recall one of my patients, Claire, who was adamant that it was only after her partner started to improve his diet, too, that she started to see results on the scales. Sounds too good to be true? With my scientific hat on, it's more likely that Claire's success was the result of the increased support from her partner and the fewer temptations she was exposed to at home rather than the change in her partner's oral microbes. But that said, the fact that our oral microbiota has been linked to weight gain does pose an interesting thought – and if nothing else, it may encourage your partner to also add a few extra portions of plants into their diet.

For those of you who haven't yet met, say hello to your GM . . .

On the face of it, our gut microbes appear quite simple, really, just living their single cellular existence. However, it's all just an act. They are, in fact, incredibly smart, which is why you'll find them not randomly scattered but instead strategically located along the gut with other like-minded microbes, forming complex and distinct ecosystems adapted to their environment. There are four key concepts about our GM that are worth knowing.

1. THE BASICS: **not just bacteria**

When I talk about the GM, I'm not just referring to bacteria but also to other types of microbes such as fungi and viruses which live in our gut too. The fungi component is known as our mycobiota, and the virus component as the virome. Although they also play a role in health and disease, our understanding of their function is still at a very early stage, unlike their bacterial counterparts, where more of their functions have been mapped out, giving us a fair idea of how they go about their daily business. What's even more striking is that some parasites (yes, they live in the gut too) are said to be more common in healthy people. Those with gut issues such as irritable bowel syndrome (IBS) and inflammatory bowel disease (IBD) have been shown to have less, suggesting that some parasites may indeed play a protective role.

2. THE BASICS: **the goal is diversity**

Generally speaking, a higher level of GM diversity is associated with better overall health. The more diverse your GM, the greater the breadth of skills your GM 'team' possesses. So just like any football team, the most successful isn't the one with all super-star strikers but the one with a range of skills to provide balance. Having a more diverse GM also increases our resilience to infection. It's similar to a thriving garden: if you have all the same type of plants and a certain disease comes along, it could wipe out your entire garden. In comparison, if you have a diverse range of plants, it is very unlikely that one disease has the right array of 'weapons' to wipe them all out – some will naturally be resistant. The same goes for your GM.

3. THE BASICS: no single ideal GM

No two people have the same GM. Even identical twins house their own unique GM. When people talk about the GM, they often use the terms 'microbiota' and 'microbiome' interchangeably. But there is a crucial difference. The term 'microbiota' refers to the actual community of microbial cells (e.g. bacteria). It is all the genes within these cells that determine what they're capable of doing and how they interact with human cells, and this is what we call the 'microbiome'. Different microbiotas (groups of microbes) can share similar microbiomes (sets of genes). This leads us to the incredible and fascinating fact that different microbes can perform similar tasks; for example, there are many different bacteria that can produce B vitamins. Therefore, up to a point, many microbes are interchangeable in terms of what they can do for us. Another 'm' term I feel it's appropriate to bring in at this point is the microbial 'metabolome'. This is just a fancy science term used to describe the tangible output of what the microbes produce, for example, vitamins and other chemicals. This metabolome is the key to understanding what the microbiota is actually doing. With that in mind, while there is no ideal microbiota, there is a health-associated microbiota for every person, meaning there is an optimal GM that's just right for you. If you look after your GM with plenty of plant-based foods, by practising mindfulness and sleeping well, among other strategies we'll discuss, chances are you'll cultivate your own optimal GM.

4. THE BASICS: good versus bad

Often, microbes are referred to as good or bad. But just like most people, the behaviour of any one microbe can be good or bad depending on the environment it finds itself in. Think about yourself: if you've had a poor night's sleep or are so hungry you've reached 'hangry' (hunger expressed as anger), then, despite being a genuinely good person, I'm sure you can get a little grumpy. It turns out our microbes are just like us. For example, *Clostridioides difficile* (*C. diff*) infection claims thousands of lives in Western countries each year, yet around 3 per cent of healthy adults (and 66 per cent of babies) have *C. diff* living in their gut. It's only when *C. diff* 'acts out' and overgrows, typically in people with weak immunity, that it starts to produce toxins triggering diarrhoea and, in severe cases, fever, gut inflammation and nausea.

What can it do for me?

Now that we have the more formal introductions out of the way, it's time to get down to business and discuss what our GM is actually doing for us. On a day-to-day basis, what are we getting from these guys? To answer this, I have put together a snapshot of the GM's basic skillset. You can think of it as your GM's CV. When reviewing this, it's worth remembering that CVs are based on your track record, so to speak. This means that there's no guarantee your GM will continue achieving at such a high level going forward if things – for example, your lifestyle – aren't supportive. Of course, if you, as a kind and motivating boss, continue to create a nice 'working' environment, there's a strong chance your GM will continue its high-level output. On the flip side, if it's overworked and underpaid, then its productivity is likely to take a nosedive.

Our GM and response to medication

Ever wondered why your response to a medication may be different to other people's? Although genetics play a key role (between 20 per cent and 95 per cent, depending on the medication), so does our GM. In fact, different microbes can do different things to medications, including activating or deactivating them, and even converting some into harmful waste products. The latter mechanism is thought to explain, at least in part, why only a subset of people experience severe diarrhoea following common colon-cancer chemotherapies and gut-lining damage after taking anti-inflammatory drugs such as ibuprofen. Our GM may also explain the variable response to certain types of cancer therapies. Indeed, one study found that a more diverse GM was linked to better response to an immune-system therapy in melanoma patients.

If you take regular medication, you may be wondering at this point which microbes you need to improve your success rates and therefore what diet you should be following. Those are the ultimate questions, and ones which hundreds of researchers around the world, including my research group, are working to answer. In the meantime, nurturing your GM with the strategies outlined in the pages to come is considered the best place to start.

Gut Microbiota's curriculum vitae (CV)

- *Can make vitamins (e.g. vitamin K and B vitamins), amino acids (protein building blocks), hormones (e.g. noradrenaline), chemical messengers (e.g. serotonin) and many others.*

- *Trains our immune system.*

- *Produces important molecules that strengthen the gut barrier and may help balance blood sugar, lower blood fats, regulate appetite, facilitate communication with the brain and ultimately help prevent against many diseases.*

- *Communicates with our other vital organs, including our brain, liver and heart.*

- *Prevents invasion from bad microbes.*

- *Enjoys eating fibre and antioxidants from plants.*

- *Metabolizes drugs and deactivates toxins.*

- *Influences gut movement and function.*

Assessment: HOW DIVERSE IS YOUR GM?

There are many factors known to affect your GM. Some of them we can change, or at least influence, such as diet (a modifiable factor), and others we can't, such as our age (an unmodifiable factor). The empowering thing about our GM is that so much of it is modifiable – in fact, it turns out that our environment has more of an effect on our GM than our genetics. Targeting our diet is one of the most effective ways we can boost our GM diversity. Most of the research done so far has found that people with high-fibre diets from a wide range of plant-based foods have greater diversity. So let's begin by looking at how much fibre, plant-based diversity and additional GM-loving foods you're getting, using the diet assessments at www.TheGutHealthDoctor.com.

Central to health and well-being

It's easy to understand how our GM can impact the rest of our gut health, given its close proximity. But it's a little harder to visualize how it could possibly impact other organs that are further afield, like our brain. Thankfully, this concept isn't one we simply need to leave to faith (I am a scientist, after all), as there is mounting scientific evidence that demonstrates just how our GM and our other organs interact with each other.

In the past few years we've come to understand, at least in part, three of the communication styles that our GM tends to use:

1. THE IMMUNE SYSTEM (think house alarm)

2. THE NERVOUS SYSTEM (think mobile phone)

3. THE CIRCULATION, that is, the blood and lymphatic system (think postal service)

Our GM makes full use of each of these, depending on the type of message it wants to send and how quickly it wants to send it. For example, if it's something urgent, like a viral invasion, then it's more likely to pick up the mobile or trigger the alarm to alert the rest of the body rather than relying on 'snail mail'. However, if it's something slow and gradual, such as a chronic disease, then sending packages via the postal service is often used. To date, an unbalanced (often called dysbiotic) GM has been linked with over 70 different conditions. But research is still only in its early stages, meaning we still don't know whether the altered GM contributes to disease (GM is the driver, disease is the passenger) or whether it's the other way around.

INSIDE THE BODY

1

IMMUNE CELLS
(the immune system)

2

NERVES
(the nervous system)

3

BLOOD VESSELS
(the circulation)

INSIDE
THE GUT

**INTESTINAL
WALL CELLS**

**GUT
MICROBES**

**METABOLITES
FROM MICROBES**

Despite this, after ten years working as a clinician, I'm convinced that everyone can benefit from looking after their GM, whether it directly or indirectly impacts on a specific condition or not. So, even if you're suffering from a condition where the evidence is still limited in terms of the role of the GM, which is indeed most areas, why not give some of the simple, cost-effective diet strategies in Chapter 3 a go (alongside any necessary medical treatment, of course)? It's best to try out the diet strategies for a four-week period and then assess whether you notice an improvement. What do you have to lose?

Gut–brain axis

The constant, two-way communication that occurs between our gut and our brain is referred to as the gut–brain axis. The latest evidence suggests that tapping into our gut–brain axis could play a pivotal role in our mental health. With one in four of us predicted to experience a mental-health event this year alone, our gut health really is something more of us should be taking into consideration.

Although the science behind the gut–brain axis (particularly how our GM is involved) is relatively new, the 'gut feeling' phenomenon is something we've all experienced. In fact, long before science connected the two, we were using gut functions to describe our feelings and emotions: 'I've got butterflies in my stomach'; 'You don't have the guts for it'; 'I can't stomach that behaviour'... clearly our ancestors were on to something.

Our understanding of the connection between our brain and our GM is still in the early stages, but there is some promising evidence building. Trials have shown not only that our GM is implicated in our mental health but that by modifying our GM with the simple diet strategies discussed in Chapter 3 and the recipes in Chapter 8, we can help manage mental-health conditions such as depression (alongside medication and therapy, as needed). What's more, by nourishing our GM with both the diet and non-diet strategies discussed in the chapters to come, we may even be able to prevent some cases of depression and anxiety.

In my practice I have witnessed the powerful role diet can play in the management of some people's mental health, including that of twenty-four-year-old Paul. When Paul first walked into my room at the clinic, his shoulders were hunched, his head down, his voice soft and his words mumbled; it was clear he was going through a tough time. As Paul and I got talking, he opened up about his history of depression, which first started after moving away for university at the age of twenty-one. He described himself as having been very sociable before that – he'd been captain of the football team and dated his high-school sweetheart – but by the age of twenty-two, he explained, 'I'd lost all interest in life.' He'd stopped playing sport, broken up with his girlfriend and distanced himself from his close friends. He saw his family GP three times over the summer and was prescribed an antidepressant. Although initially hesitant, Paul decided to give the antidepressant a go as he headed back to university. Over the following three months he noticed some improvement in his mood, although he still found himself avoiding social events. As fate would have it, Paul just so happened to be in the waiting room of his university GP when he stumbled upon an article I'd written describing one of my favourite clinical trials: the SMILES trial. The article really resonated with Paul, who moments later found himself explaining to his GP that, although he had come in with a plan to consider increasing his dose of antidepressants, he had just read a convincing article supporting the role of diet, so for now wanted to hold off until he'd had time to look into this further. With his GP's approval, two weeks later, Paul was sitting in front of me with a rather novel request; he wanted to follow the study I'd written about in that article. So that's exactly what we did. Paul filled out the assessment questionnaires that had been used in the study and I counselled him on the Mediterranean diet, just as the dietitian had done with the participants in the SMILES trial. The diet was high in wholegrains, vegetables, fruit, nuts, seeds, legumes and extra virgin olive oil, and contained nearly three times the dietary fibre most of us eat (as we'll discuss in Chapter 3). I reviewed Paul six times over the following twelve weeks, as they had in the study. I'm not going to paint a false picture and say it was easy. It certainly wasn't. Paul was going from a heavily fast-food-based diet to eating home-made, mostly plant-based meals. At each phone review Paul talked me through the tough days when he'd end up paying a visit to those devilishly tempting golden arches, and together we troubleshot (which included using some quick and easy recipes) and moved forward (we didn't dwell on those tough days). Now, I'm a big believer in diet, but when Paul walked back into clinic twelve weeks later, sporting the biggest smile, from ear to ear, the colour back in his face and with a strong posture, even I was impressed. His first words – 'Megan, life is good' – pretty much summed it up for Paul. I received an email from him nine months later. Paul shared his mum's gratitude with me, and his family GP's decision to lower his antidepressant dose with the goal of stopping them altogether if things continued going to plan. And for those romantics out there, Paul added that he'd also rekindled his relationship with his high-school sweetheart.

Assessment: HOW HAPPY ARE YOU?

This is such an important question, but one that too few of us ask ourselves. So, let's take a look at your current happiness levels using a validated questionnaire.

When completing this assessment, it's best not to take too long thinking about each question. The first answer that comes into your head is probably the right one for you. If you find some of the questions difficult, give the answer that is true for you most of the time. Head over to www.TheGutHealthDoctor.com to complete the happiness assessment.

Doing damage

The impact of our lifestyle on our GM is not always positive. Sometimes it just takes a moment for us to stop and reflect on the way we treat our bodies (and therefore our microbes), to realize that perhaps we haven't been the best hosts – after all, they've been looking out for us, but have we been looking out for them?

Without intending to bring on 'friend-guilt', but rather to help strengthen your relationship, let's take a look at some of our GM's key vulnerabilities. In doing so, next time you're considering a certain behaviour, perhaps you'll spare a thought to how it may also affect your microbes.

1. Medication

There is growing awareness that antibiotics (which translates to 'anti-life' in Greek) not only kill the overgrown and 'bad' bacteria but also harm the beneficial guys. In some people these changes appear to be irreversible, meaning not all the good guys repopulate after the antibiotics. It's not just antibiotics we need to watch out for either – a recent study has suggested that over a quarter of non-antibiotic medications (of the more than 900 tested) can potentially impact the growth of our gut microbes.

Don't get me wrong, medications such as antibiotics are incredibly important, but the next time your GP explains that they may not be necessary because your infection is likely to be viral in origin (which means antibiotics won't work), it's worth taking them seriously. Similarly, if you're taking medication because it's easier than changing your lifestyle, for example decreasing your alcohol intake in the case of reflux, or relying on sleeping pills instead of working on your sleep hygiene (check out page 164 for this), then it might be worth having a rethink of the potential harm you could be doing. That said, don't go getting too hasty – any decision regarding changing medication should be done under guidance from your health-care team.

It's not all doom and gloom when it comes to our microbes and medication. One of the most common medications prescribed for type 2 diabetes (known as metformin) has recently been shown to benefit our GM. This discovery is thought to be a new mechanism by which metformin improves millions of patients' blood-sugar regulation. And it's likely not alone, with several other medications suspected to target the GM in order to exert their medicinal benefit.

2. Sleep

Sleep disturbance, including both shift work and jet lag, is another major factor shown to disrupt our GM. This is because, like us, our GM exhibits a sleep–wake cycle, known as the circadian rhythm. Interestingly, the negative impact of sleep disturbance on our GM may explain, at least in part, the increased risk of weight gain and diabetes in people with disturbed sleep. Further still, research suggests that this relationship is bidirectional. This means that a disturbed GM may also lead to disturbed sleep. There is some good news, however. One study showed that a type of probiotic improved sleep in a group of students, compared to placebo (a fake probiotic). In my practice, I've also found that simple dietary changes to boost our GM have helped many shift-workers improve their sleep quality. In turn, working on your sleep hygiene may also be worth a thought to ensure that not just you but your GM, too, get the most out of pillow time.

For those frequent fliers, particularly on long-haul flights, and who also suffer with gut issues, check out page 149 for some pre-flight nutrition tips for your gut.

3. Dieting

What about that crazy diet you may have tried last summer – did that impact your GM? Interestingly, although our GM can change within days of being on an extreme diet, the overall changes that occur to the microbes following a short-term diet are not as extreme as you may think. What does happen, however, is that it alters the function of these microbes, that is, what the microbes actually do and what they produce (the metabolome). Animal research suggests that the rapid weight-regain phenomenon that occurs with 'yo-yo' dieting (you know, when you seem to regain the weight in half the time it took you to lose it) may in fact be down to our GM. The study not only demonstrated that mice with a previous 'weight gain, weight loss' cycle were more susceptible to fast weight gain the second time around, it also showed that this tendency to gain more weight could be transferred to other mice via a poop transplant. This finding suggests that the weight gain was because of their GM and not because of other factors like the mouse's metabolism. Now, before the 'Oh no, what have I done?' feeling sets in, the researchers did also show that this tendency to regain weight rapidly could be reversed with the right nutrition (we'll discuss this in Chapter 3).

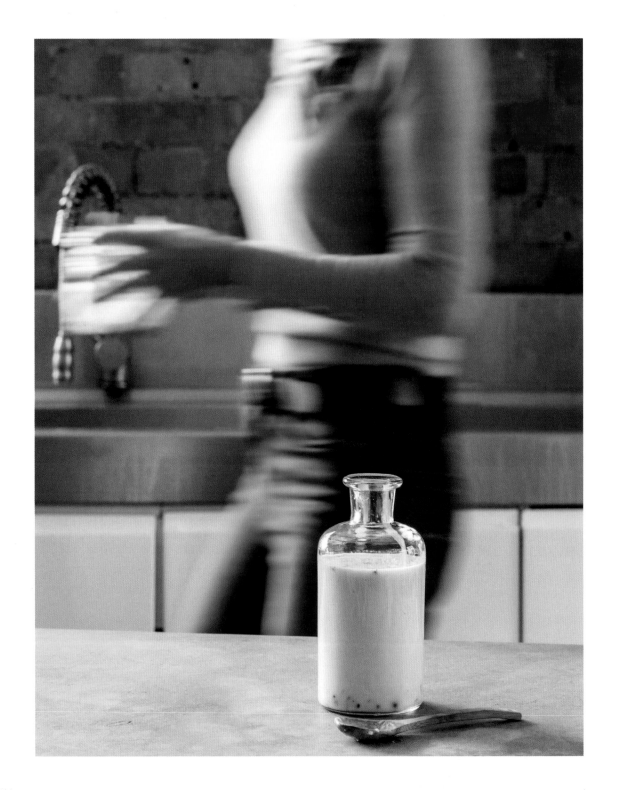

Checklist for looking after your GM

○ PLANT-BASED DIET DIVERSITY (SEE PAGE 60)

○ SPEND MORE TIME OUTDOORS AMONG NATURE

○ MOVE YOUR BODY OFTEN (SEE PAGE 180)

○ OPT FOR A PROBIOTIC IN SPECIFIC CASES (SEE PAGE 54)

○ CONSIDER A FURRY PET (CONDITIONS APPLY*)

○ AVOID YO-YO DIETING

○ DON'T IGNORE GUT SYMPTOMS (SEE PAGE 81)

○ BOOST YOUR SLEEP QUALITY (SEE PAGE 164)

○ REDUCE YOUR STRESS LEVELS (SEE PAGE 168)

○ AVOID UNNECESSARY MEDICATIONS AND DON'T SMOKE

○ TRY FERMENTED FOODS (SEE PAGE 56)

○ BE SENSIBLE WITH ALCOHOL (NO MORE THAN TWO STANDARD DRINKS A DAY)

* Although research has linked furry pets with better immunity, keep in mind that pets need a lot of love and attention. If you're not up for it, just play with your neighbour's.

CHAPTER 3

Nutrition for the gut

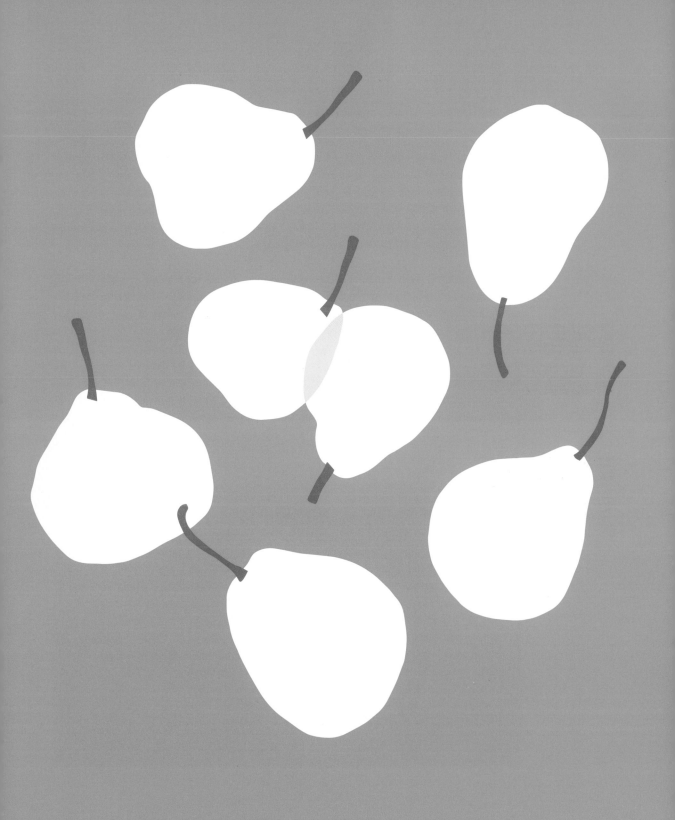

Nutrition for the gut

It was during my PhD when I had my first ever 'light-bulb moment' – one of those moments that can fundamentally alter your understanding of something. In this case, it was my understanding of nutrition. I was analysing my patients' food diaries when it dawned on me that our view of nutrition is pretty self-centred. Meal times have always been about feeding ourselves – what do we want? What do we feel like eating? We rarely spare a thought for the trillions of microbes that look after us on a daily basis.

Until very recently, even the scientific community has viewed food solely through the lens of its impact on the human metabolism, forgetting completely about our gut microbiota (GM) metabolism. The consequences have included some pretty drastic changes to our food supply, the biggest one being the creation of what is now known as the 'Western diet'.

Traditionally, it was thought that fibre had no perceived nutritional benefit. As it can't be digested by human cells, it was regarded as waste and used for animal feed (bet they had great gut health!). Indeed, refined grains like white bread were, historically, considered of higher quality and as a marker of wealth, up until the late twentieth century. Thankfully, that

The Western diet

It's been implicated in just about every chronic disease. It's characterized by excess calories, high intakes of processed meats, sugary desserts, refined grains and high amounts of salt (think that stereotypical fast-food meal). We haven't always eaten like that; there was a time when we had to grow and hunt our own food and make everything from scratch. But then the Industrial Revolution happened, from around the second half of the eighteenth century, and spread from Britain to other parts of the Western world. This was the start of the downward spiral, although, at the time, the changes were thought to reflect wealth and prosperity. Food preparation moved from people's kitchens on to manufacturing lines, processed food was in, wholefood was out and, as a result, daily fibre intakes plummeted and intakes of added sugar soared. Although originating in the geographical Western world, the diet has infiltrated much of the globe, alongside the increasing industrialization of countries in the developing world.

idea has since been dismissed, although, unfortunately, the popularity of refined grains has persisted. Similarly, the recent rise in many food additives, such as artificial sweeteners, which, because they're not absorbed in our small intestine and therefore don't 'enter' our body and directly affect human cells, have been deemed safe to consume. Fast-forward to our current understanding: we now appreciate that the nutrition we deliver to our microbes also plays a key role in our health and happiness.

This chapter is about rebalancing our perspective of nutrition by giving some well-deserved focus to feeding our microbes. But before we get into the real detail, let's set ourselves up by changing gear slightly and addressing any of those feelings of anxiety, stress or even guilt which, for so many, surround the words 'food' and 'nutrition'. Perhaps start by asking yourself whether, heading into this chapter, you were already thinking, I wonder if I have been eating right? or Are my favourite foods going to be banned? If so, I want you to get right up out of your chair, bed or wherever you may be, and then I want you to shake off those negative thoughts. Yes, that's right, I mean physically shake those shoulders and wiggle those hips. Let those negative feelings go. I know it sounds a bit absurd, but, guys, give it a try – physically letting go of unhelpful thoughts is more powerful than you might think (something we'll discuss more in Chapter 7). The fact is that nutrition is not black or white and, in my opinion, it shouldn't take precedence over the amazing flavours and feeling of community that come with eating and feeding your gut microbes. Food should be tasty, and it should be fun. Eating should be a happy experience; it shouldn't be crushed by those unhelpful thoughts, which is, sadly, something I see all too often.

One of my patients, Emily, knew all too well about the consequence of losing sight of the joy of eating. I first met Emily in my clinic six months after she'd moved away from home to start her beauty-therapy training. Emily had come to see me about her weight, which she described as 'out of control'. She explained, 'I only have to look at food and I gain weight these days.' Emily had heard that gut inflammation was linked to weight gain and was convinced this was the cause of hers. I asked Emily to describe both her current diet and her diet six months earlier, when she lived at home. Emily explained that she was from a family of cooks and had always loved her food but believed that she was now paying the price for her love of fresh pasta and home-made cheese with her 'inflamed' gut and resulting weight gain. Emily's current diet excluded all wheat, dairy and foods she'd read were high in sugar; instead she ate gluten-free products, coconut oil and vegan energy balls. When I asked her if she missed her old way of eating, she was quick to reply, 'Every day! I find myself craving fresh pasta several times a week. But I know it's bad for me and I want to look after myself.' At this point, it was clear that the only way forward was to challenge some of the nutrition information Emily had heard. I started by explaining to Emily the basic functions of the gut (as we covered in Chapter 1). This indirectly called into question several nutritional claims she had heard, for instance, the concept that sugar (specifically the common sugar, sucrose) was bad for her GM. I showed her a diagram in an old textbook that indicated where the sugar was absorbed (in the top part of the intestine, except in very rare disorders) and explained that the small amount of sugar she had been eating was unlikely to be getting into her large intestine. Therefore, the sugar itself wasn't 'harming' her GM. Instead, by restricting certain foods, such as her mum's bran cookies, which, yes, contained some sugar but also significant amounts of dietary fibre, on the whole she had in fact cut down on the very nutrient that was nourishing her GM. I could see Emily starting to realize that perhaps what she'd heard wasn't all that accurate.

Towards the end of our consultation I felt that I'd earned enough trust to propose something a little radical: for four weeks, I wanted Emily to go back to her old way of eating. That meant cooking everything from scratch, including fresh pasta (cooked al dente – I describe why on page 212), enjoying fermented dairy and even having some of her mum's bran cookies. I also encouraged her to eat more of her meals with friends and family rather than eating alone. I could see her hesitation. But I stood by the challenge, reassuring her that I was confident her weight would not increase. Four weeks later, Emily was sitting in front of me, her weight down and her food-related quality of life up.

Why was I so confident that refocusing on the enjoyment of food would work for Emily? After initially eyeballing Emily's diet during our first consultation I could see that she was not only eating much larger portions of energy-dense foods than when she was living at home with her mum (something I commonly see when people deprive themselves of favourite foods), she was also eating around 50 per cent less fibre. Emily's case is the perfect example of how, despite good intentions, losing sight of the pleasures and feeling of community associated with eating can lead unexpectedly to negative consequences.

The good news is that nourishing your GM certainly doesn't require a strict diet, nor does it mean you have to give up the enjoyment of food. In fact, part of the community feel of eating together includes feeding them, all 40 trillion of them. When it comes to nutrition for your GM, it's actually pretty simple: it's just about being aware of some of the basics, like your GM's major likes and dislikes, which, I'd argue, is common courtesy, really. Think about it: would you invite your vegan or vegetarian friends over for dinner and offer only meat? Of course not! So why would we not cater for our closest friends, the ones living inside our gut which keep guard

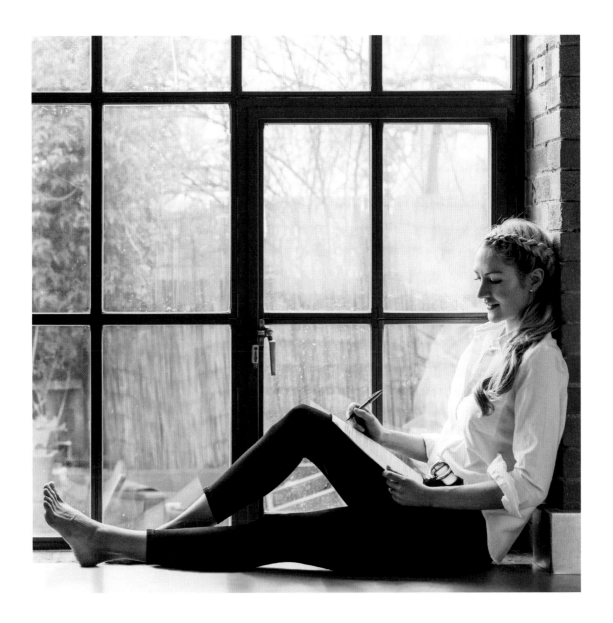

24/7? It's common sense. For those after more of a scientific incentive, if you learn how to create a diet that is varied, delicious and keeps your GM happy, the research suggests that you will soon see the benefits, and these go beyond kicking pesky gut symptoms, to increasing your ability to fight the flu, your happiness levels, your metabolism, and even the health of other organs, such as your heart and your liver (your main detoxing organ).

Food in a nutshell

Food is essentially made up of three types of macronutrients: carbohydrates, proteins and fats. These are called MACROnutrients because they are present in large amounts, unlike MICROnutrients, that is, vitamins and minerals, which are present in only very small amounts. Both macro- and micronutrients are considered essential in our diet, but they're not the only beneficial things in food. Many prebiotics and polyphenols (we'll touch on them in more detail in the pages to come) are considered food bioactives, indicating that they play an active role in our health but are not essential for basic functioning.

It's important to be aware that, at the end of the day, we eat whole foods and not single nutrients. For example, although most people refer to bread as a carbohydrate, it still contains some protein and fat. Foods are never black and white, despite our attempts to simplify and categorize them. Understanding the basics of food can help explain the big picture of diet, as well as safeguard you against the many diet myths out there (e.g. that carb-free diets are good for your gut). With this in mind, we will start off by discussing single components of food but will then tie it all together with a focus on the overall big picture of what we eat.

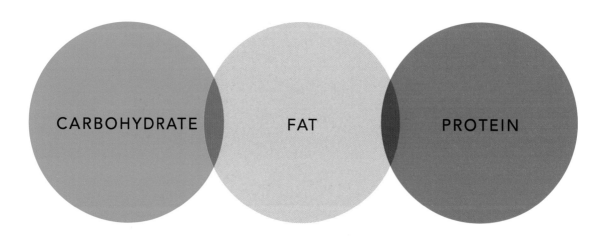

CARBOHYDRATE   FAT   PROTEIN

Macronutrients

Generally speaking, macronutrients need to be broken down into their basic building blocks before they can be absorbed from our digestive tract into our circulation: carbohydrates are broken down into sugars, proteins into amino acids and fat into fatty acids. This is the process of digestion, and different enzymes are required to break apart different types of macronutrients.

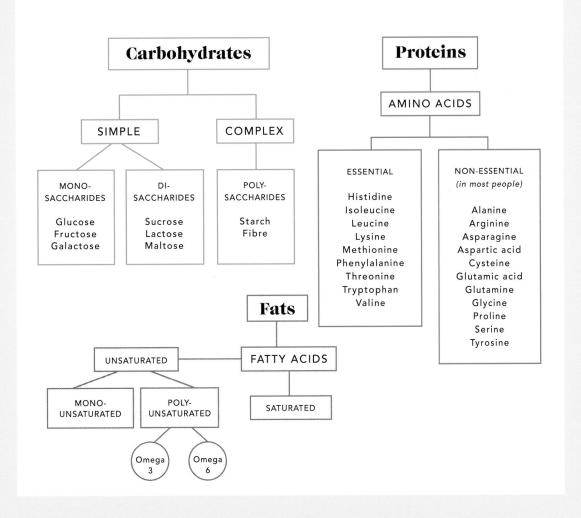

Dietary fibre

Unlike the other types of carbohydrates (yes, fibre is a type of carbohydrate), fibre isn't broken down in the small intestine. This is because humans don't make the enzymes needed to digest it, as we touched on in Chapter 1. Instead, dietary fibre continues on its merry way down the digestive tract into the large intestine, where our hungry GM eagerly awaits. I think of dietary fibre as Mother Nature's unique gift to our GM, but don't worry, we're not missing out; we get our share of the presents, as it's a mutually beneficial 'transaction'. Our helpful gut microbes have the skillset to break down many different fibres, found in food, producing a range of beneficial compounds known as short-chain fatty acids (SCFA). There are three main SCFAs you may come across: acetate, propionate and butyrate. These SCFAs are like an overachieving friend – just hearing about all the things they get up to makes you feel tired. As well as providing fuel for our gut lining, they help 'get things moving' in the large intestine, contribute to the balance of blood sugars (they can trigger cells lining the intestine to make glucose, which, essentially, tells our brain that we are full), they can stimulate our immune system and the release of gut hormones, and are also known to directly impact fat tissue, the liver and even our brain!

The benefits of fibre don't stop there: it goes beyond simply feeding our microbes. It uses its unique physical properties to: a) contribute to bulking out our poop – remember, from the 'Checking in with your poop' assessment in Chapter 1, a bulky poop is a good thing; b) thicken the contents of our gut, giving the gut muscles more to work with and regulating our pooping habits; and c) bind to other compounds, which can help prevent blood-sugar spikes and lower cholesterol levels.

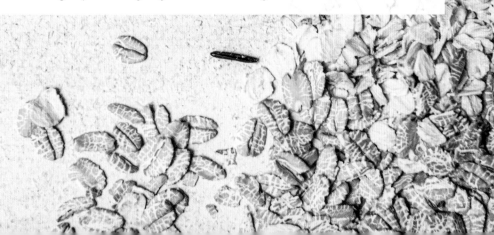

Where do we find it?

It's certainly no coincidence that fibre is found in the foods associated with the best health outcomes – that is, fibre is essentially the backbone of plant-based foods. Each plant-based food group (i.e. wholegrains, legumes, vegetables, fruits, nuts and seeds) contains different types of fibres – in fact there are thought to be over 100 different types. This explains why getting fibre from different foods within each of these groups is associated with the best overall health outcomes – yet another example of why diversity is key. But what if you're considering cutting out one of these groups, by going grain-free, for instance? Remember: One of my key rules is that your dietary choices are completely yours – no judgement to be found in the pages of this book. But I do want to share with you an unbiased view of the science, because a choice is only a real choice if it is an informed one.

When it comes to fibre from wholegrains, there is some pretty convincing evidence for its role not just in gut health but also in reducing your chances of developing several diseases, including diabetes, heart disease and several cancers. In fact, according to one study involving close to 16,000 women, fibre from wholegrains was linked with a lower risk of breast cancer, whereas fibre from vegetables and fruit didn't seem to have this benefit. This enhanced protection linked with wholegrain fibre, in contrast to other fibre sources, has also been suggested in other diseases, such as colon cancer. Further, another study, this time with over 400,000 participants, found that those with the highest consumption of wholegrains, compared to the lowest, had a reduced risk of heart issues of over 20 per cent. Now, this certainly doesn't mean you should be prioritizing wholegrain fibre above all else, because plant-based foods are more than just fibre, they're densely packed with vitamins, minerals, polyphenols and other bioactive components. However, what it does highlight is that getting fibre from each food group is worth giving some serious thought to.

How much do you need?

As a general guide, when it comes to getting in your gut-boosting fibres, the evidence suggests that adults should be aiming for at least two pieces of fruit, five portions of vegetables, three portions of wholegrains and one to two portions from nuts, seeds or legumes each day. For those into number-crunching, this will generally deliver around 30 grams of fibre, which is in line with most national fibre recommendations for adults. I know this may sound like a lot, particularly with vegetables, but as you'll see in Chapter 8, we've got it covered, with most of the main meal recipes providing three portions of vegetable and close to 10 grams of fibre per portion. For those wanting to up their fibre intake even further, please go right ahead. There is research that supports that going beyond 30 grams per day further lowers your risks of chronic disease like type 2 diabetes, heart disease and depression; the SMILES trial from Chapter 2 provided 50g/day. But before you get too heavy-handed with your fibre portions, check out my tips for the best way to increase your fibre intake on pages 50–51.

Lowering your risk

I get that for many, making long-term changes to their diet can take a little more convincing. So here are some hard stats that I've often used with my family and friends. A powerful study has demonstrated that even small increases in fibre can have a big impact on our health. A paper published in the *Lancet* (one of the top science journals) pooled together the evidence from millions of people and found that an increase of 8 grams of fibre per day was linked with:

- 19% ⬇ **RISK OF HEART DISEASE**

- 15% ⬇ **RISK OF TYPE 2 DIABETES**

- 8% ⬇ **RISK OF COLON CANCER**

- 7% ⬇ **RISK OF DEATH FROM ALL CAUSES**

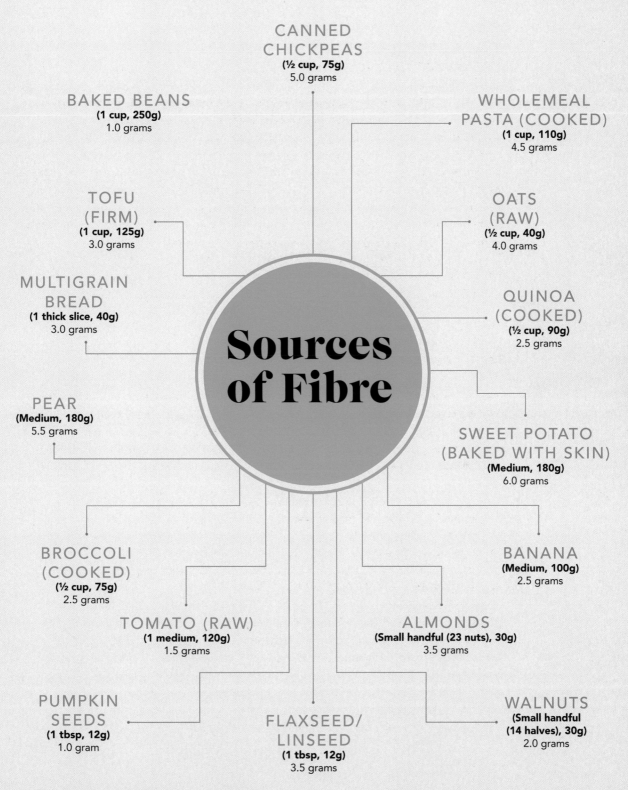

Sources of Fibre

CANNED CHICKPEAS
(½ cup, 75g)
5.0 grams

BAKED BEANS
(1 cup, 250g)
1.0 grams

WHOLEMEAL PASTA (COOKED)
(1 cup, 110g)
4.5 grams

TOFU (FIRM)
(1 cup, 125g)
3.0 grams

OATS (RAW)
(½ cup, 40g)
4.0 grams

MULTIGRAIN BREAD
(1 thick slice, 40g)
3.0 grams

QUINOA (COOKED)
(½ cup, 90g)
2.5 grams

PEAR
(Medium, 180g)
5.5 grams

SWEET POTATO (BAKED WITH SKIN)
(Medium, 180g)
6.0 grams

BROCCOLI (COOKED)
(½ cup, 75g)
2.5 grams

BANANA
(Medium, 100g)
2.5 grams

TOMATO (RAW)
(1 medium, 120g)
1.5 grams

ALMONDS
(Small handful (23 nuts), 30g)
3.5 grams

PUMPKIN SEEDS
(1 tbsp, 12g)
1.0 gram

FLAXSEED/ LINSEED
(1 tbsp, 12g)
3.5 grams

WALNUTS
(Small handful (14 halves), 30g)
2.0 grams

Source: USDA Food Composition Database.

The practical stuff

As you can see, fibre really does deserve a prominent place on our plate. So, what constitutes a portion of fibre-rich food? Not to get fanatical about measuring food – I certainly don't recommend weighing your meals – but having a general idea of what constitutes a portion is helpful. So here it is:

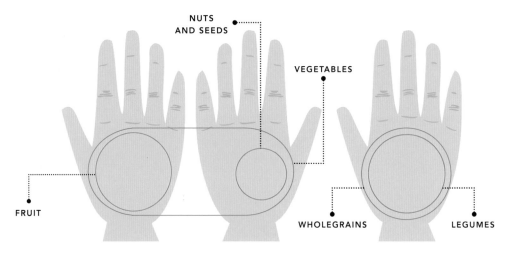

NUTS AND SEEDS

VEGETABLES

FRUIT

WHOLEGRAINS

LEGUMES

WHEN IT COMES TO INCREASING THE AMOUNT OF PLANT-BASED FOODS IN OUR DIET, THERE ARE THREE THINGS WORTH KNOWING:

1 INCREASE SLOW AND GRADUALLY:

It takes our large intestine time to adjust and adapt to the increased 'load'. If you go from little to a lot of fibre too quickly, your GM may get a little carried away (think post-diet binge), leaving your gut feeling a little bloated, and probably gassy too. To avoid this, start by increasing your intake by one portion per day, after one week add another portion and continue this gradual pattern of weekly increases until you've reached your target. If your gut is a little on the sensitive side, you might like to start a little more slowly, increasing by half a portion each time.

2 DON'T FORGET TO HYDRATE:

Generally speaking, fibre needs water to work some of its magic. With this in mind, consider adding an extra glass of water or two as you increase your fibre-rich foods.

3 MAKE THEM IRRESISTIBLE:

Changing habits can be hard at the best of times, so help yourself out and 'dress up' your plant-based foods with tasty flavour combos. We'll be doing plenty of this in Chapter 8.

12 ways to boost your fibre intake

1

Add flavour and texture to your favourite soup by stirring in cooked barley or legumes.

2

Sprinkle mixed seeds on your breakfast – whether it's cereal, toast or eggs, it's always a winner.

3

Love lasagne? Why not replace a third of the mince with cooked lentils for a twist your GM will love too?

4

Don't waste your time or fibre – keep the skin on your fruit and vegetables.

5

Baking muffins? Replace one third of the flour with quick oats.

6

Up the fibre in your next fry-up with a portion of beans and grilled tomato.

7

Add low-sugar granola to your yoghurt – a delicious crunch with no cooking necessary.

8

Boost your Bolognese sauce by adding lentils or legumes, or by grating in onion, carrots and courgettes.

9

Making meatballs? Replace a third of the mince with uncooked oats, lentils or legumes.

10

In a rush? Frozen vegetables are a convenient and nutritious addition to any meal.

11

Banish those hungry feelings with a small handful of nuts, seeds and dried fruit.

12

Make the switch from white to wholegrain and seeded bread – your GM will thank you.

Prebiotics

A PREbiotic – not to be mistaken for a PRObiotic – is essentially food that feeds specific beneficial microbes. But wait, isn't that the same as fibre? Indeed, most prebiotics are a type of dietary fibre, although not all dietary fibres are prebiotics. There are two reasons for this. Firstly, not all fibres can be eaten by our GM. Secondly, for a dietary fibre to 'win' a prebiotic title, it must prove itself (and a health benefit) in several scientific trials, meaning it really does have to work for that coveted prebiotic title.

The main prebiotics include inulin, fructo-oligosaccharides (FOS) and galacto-oligosaccharides (GOS). These are found in over 35,000 plant species, with some of the most common sources listed below. The benefits of prebiotics range from improving blood-sugar control and appetite regulation to supporting bone health and skin health. There are also a number of trials demonstrating the benefit of prebiotics on immunity, with some pretty convincing evidence that prebiotics can reduce your risk of needing antibiotics, particularly in kids and the elderly.

So, which prebiotic supplement do I recommend you take? It's simple – none. That's right: for the majority of people, taking advantage of the naturally occurring prebiotics in food is absolutely the best way to feed your GM. There are some scenarios where I do recommend supplements, but these are infrequent and to be taken on a case-by-case basis. If you are considering taking a prebiotic supplement, keep in mind that more is not always better.

Fruit	Vegetables	Grains & nuts	Others
Apricots	Artichokes	Almonds	Legumes
Dates	Asparagus	Amaranth	(black beans,
Grapefruit	Beetroot	Barley	butterbeans,
Nectarines	Brussels sprouts	Cashews	chickpeas, etc.)
Pomegranates	Chicory root	Freekeh	Chai tea
Prunes	Fennel bulb	Hazelnuts	Chamomile tea
Persimmon	Garlic	Pistachios	Dandelion tea
Watermelon	Leeks	Rye	Fennel tea
Dried figs	Okra	Spelt	Quince paste
Dried mango	Onions	Wheat berries	Silken tofu

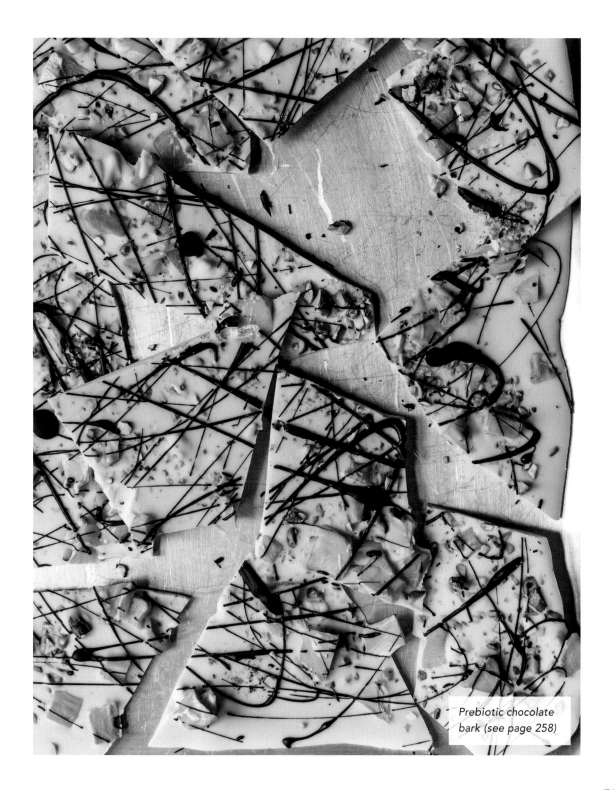

Prebiotic chocolate bark (see page 258)

Probiotics

Next up is probiotics, which is the term used to describe microbes that are good for us; they're the ones we want in our gut. Now, just like the term 'prebiotic', 'probiotic' is a title that a microbe must earn. It's also worth keeping in mind that, although most common probiotics are a type of bacteria, some are also yeast.

THERE ARE THREE MAIN CRITERIA TO FULFIL THE PROBIOTIC DEFINITION:

1. THE MICROBES HAVE TO BE ALIVE.

2. THEY HAVE TO BE PRESENT IN LARGE NUMBERS.

3. THEY HAVE TO HAVE EVIDENCE OF A HEALTH BENEFIT.

Who should take a probiotic capsule?

Generally speaking, if you're in good health, the evidence for taking a probiotic at this stage is actually pretty weak. If there is something in particular that you're aiming to manage, for example a gut symptom or a health condition, then, in some cases, it may be advisable. It all comes down to your specific condition and whether there is any evidence for a particular type of probiotic. It's also worth recognizing that different probiotics do different things and therefore have different indications. It's like medication – you wouldn't take a painkiller to improve your cholesterol. One of my patients, Hayley, is a good example of this.

Hayley came to see me after suffering for several years with IBS. Hayley had previously tried the standard dietary recommendations for IBS (we'll discuss them in Chapter 6), and although that did improve some of her symptoms, she was travelling frequently with work so she found them difficult to implement consistently. Hayley had continued living with her bothersome bloating, belly cramps and loose poops until she had an 'accident' at work. When I asked Hayley if she was taking any supplements, she explained that she'd trialled several probiotics which friends had recommended but hadn't found any that helped her. Hayley was keen to give one of the clinically backed probiotics a try. We matched the particular type of bacteria, the dose and duration, and Hayley documented her symptoms for seven days before she started taking them and then again four weeks after taking the carefully chosen probiotic.

Three weeks into Hayley's trial, I received an email from her describing the positive impact the probiotics were having, not only on her symptoms but also on her anxiety (which I saw as very much linked with her symptoms). But she wasn't just emailing about the good news; Hayley had a urinary tract infection and was prescribed antibiotics. She had taken them before and said that they'd messed with her gut so she was worried they'd undo all the good work that had come from the probiotics. I suggested that she stop taking her IBS probiotics and instead replace them with a probiotic designed specifically to help prevent antibiotic-associated gut upset (known as antibiotic-associated diarrhoea, something we'll discuss on page 94), a common side effect of antibiotics. When I saw Hayley back in the clinic two weeks later, her symptoms had continued to improve and she was thrilled to report that her antibiotics had only a minimal impact on her symptoms, unlike on previous occasions. Although Hayley acknowledged that there were still some lifestyle changes she needed to make, finding a probiotic that worked for her gave her the very confidence boost she needed to persist.

When deciding whether a probiotic is right for you, there are several things worth considering. To help simplify things, I have summarized the six steps I recommend you follow in the figure alongside. As a guide to get you started, I have developed a summary of evidence-based probiotic prescriptions: visit www.TheGutHealthDoctor.com

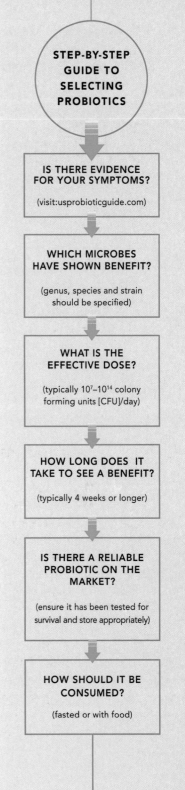

STEP-BY-STEP GUIDE TO SELECTING PROBIOTICS

IS THERE EVIDENCE FOR YOUR SYMPTOMS?

(visit:usprobioticguide.com)

WHICH MICROBES HAVE SHOWN BENEFIT?

(genus, species and strain should be specified)

WHAT IS THE EFFECTIVE DOSE?

(typically 10^7–10^{14} colony forming units [CFU]/day)

HOW LONG DOES IT TAKE TO SEE A BENEFIT?

(typically 4 weeks or longer)

IS THERE A RELIABLE PROBIOTIC ON THE MARKET?

(ensure it has been tested for survival and store appropriately)

HOW SHOULD IT BE CONSUMED?

(fasted or with food)

Fermented foods

Let me start by declaring that I am pro fermented food – the flavours, the journey and the (albeit anecdotal) health benefits associated with them have earned them a regular place in my diet. But with my science hat on, I must admit that the concept of a fermented food and its health benefits are not as straightforward as you may have hoped.

Despite their recent rise in popularity, fermented foods have been around for thousands of years. In fact, fermented food has earned a prized place in most cultures, each crafting unique flavours and traditions around the art of fermenting. Some of my favourites include: Japanese natto (soybeans), Korean kimchi (cabbage), Slavic kvass (a non-alcoholic rye drink), French crème fraîche (sour cream), Mexican pozol (a corn drink), Ethiopian injera (teff flatbread), Indian dhokla (steamed breakfast cakes), Indonesian tempeh (soybean cake), just to name a few . . .

Generally speaking, any food or drink that relies on microbes to convert simple ingredients into a final product fits the fermented-food bill. Indeed, as much as one third of our daily diet is thought to rely on the process of fermentation – bread, chocolate, cheese, yoghurt, olives, vinegar, soy sauce, coffee and even alcohol. Now, before you put the weekend's cocktail binge down to a selfless quest for good gut health, fermented doesn't automatically mean it's good for you. Similarly, not all fermented food contains live microbes. This is because many die off in the making, during processes involving heat (e.g. in the case of bread) and filtration (e.g. in the case of wine). Nonetheless, the benefits of fermented food extend beyond the live microbes. An example of this has been observed with sourdough bread: even though the microbes die off during baking, when compared to non-fermented wholewheat bread it was shown to have a better response on blood sugars. Now I must declare that this was just a single study, so not to be taken as gospel. Similarly, although not all yoghurts contain significant amounts of live microbes, in large studies yoghurt has been linked with more pronounced health benefits, including weight management, compared to unfermented dairy products such as milk.

On the whole, the scientific evidence behind fermented foods is limited at this moment in time. But this certainly shouldn't be interpreted as saying that eating fermented foods has no benefit (anecdotally speaking, I believe many do); it's just that the high-quality studies in humans haven't been done yet – something I'm passionate about changing. Health benefits aside, many traditional forms of fermented food are delicious, so why not give them a try? For a beginner's guide to making your own fermented foods, as well as the practical aspects, such as how much you should be having, head to page 264.

Potential benefits of traditional fermented foods

EACH BENEFIT IS UNIQUE TO DIFFERENT FERMENTED FOODS.

1. **CONTAIN LIVE MICROBES**
   linked with a wide range of health benefits (check out their CV on page 29).

2. **IMPROVE TASTE, TEXTURE AND DIGESTIBILITY**
   (e.g. fermentation of grape skins enhances the extraction of those gut-loving polyphenols found in red wine). Fermenting may also lower the gluten content in some sourdough breads, and lactose (milk sugar) in dairy products.

3. **CAN INCREASE CONCENTRATIONS OF VITAMINS**
   such as folate, riboflavin and B12.

4. **CONTAIN BENEFICIAL COMPOUNDS**
   such as organic acids which may help to reduce blood pressure, improve blood-sugar control and support the immune system. Brain-messenger molecules such as gamma-aminobutyric acids (GABA), which are known to have a calming effect on the brain, are also found in some fermented food.

5. **MAY REMOVE/REDUCE TOXINS AND ANTINUTRIENTS**
   (e.g. fermentation can significantly reduce phytic acid, which, although not harmful per se, can inhibit the absorption of other nutrients such as zinc, as we discuss on page 69).

Phytochemicals

Phytochemicals is just the sciencey name for a group of plant chemicals. As we touched on earlier, these are different to macronutrients (e.g. fats and protein) and micronutrients (e.g. folate and iron) because they're not essential. Instead, consider them as a way to boost your health that bit further. It's kind of like buying a new pair of trainers or new model of phone – neither is essential, but both can enhance your performance and efficiency. One of the most well-studied classes of phytochemical are the polyphenols. These include flavanols, which are linked to the health benefits of dark chocolate, and anthocyanin, which gives berries their brilliant red, purple and blue colour. The thing about polyphenols is that around 90 per cent of them are malabsorbed in the small intestine and therefore join our GM in the large intestine. This is where much of the magic is thought to happen, in that our microbes help to transform them into a range of absorbable and potentially beneficial chemicals linked with cancer prevention and better heart and mental health.

Things get even more fascinating. The benefits of polyphenols appear to be dependent on your unique GM and whether it is able to metabolize the specific polyphenol you've eaten. To follow on the idea, my colleagues at King's College London are currently investigating whether this GM-dependency may explain why some people do better on different diets.

Where can we find these health-boosters? Polyphenols are found in a wide range of plant-based foods, with some of the top sources outlined opposite. It's worth having a think about how many regularly feature in your diet. Are there any you might like to try? To get more in your diet, why not add some berries to your breakfast bowl, or put olives in your pasta sauce or hazelnuts on your salad? For those tempted to reach for the supplement instead, in most cases, the food sources are linked with the best health outcomes.

We often forget the power of herbs and spices, but not only do they add even more polyphenols to your diet, they can seriously boost the flavour of your meals. You might like to experiment with the top polyphenol-containing seasonings on the opposite page.

Top polyphenol foods

- **DRINKS**
  Filtered coffee, black tea, red wine, green tea, cocoa

- **FRUIT**
  Black chokeberry, black elderberry, blueberry, blackcurrant, plum, cherry, blackberry, strawberry, raspberry, prune, black grapes, apple

- **NUTS AND SEEDS**
  Flaxseed, chestnuts, hazelnuts, pecans, almonds

- **VEGETABLES AND LEGUMES**
  Black olives, green olives, globe artichoke heads, roasted soybeans, chicory, red onion, spinach, black beans, white beans, broccoli, asparagus

- **FATS**
  Extra virgin olive oil, rapeseed oil

Top fifteen herbs & spices			
	• CAPERS	• OREGANO	• BASIL
	• CELERY SEEDS	• PEPPERMINT	• CURRY POWDER
	• CLOVES	• ROSEMARY	• GINGER
	• SAGE	• SPEARMINT	• CINNAMON
	• THYME	• STAR ANISE	• CARAWAY

Derived from 100 Richest dietary sources of polyphenols published in the European Journal of Clinical Nutrition. *(Ranked per 100g.) Values can differ between crops.*

Plant-based diet diversity

According to the United Nations, 75 per cent of plant diversity has been lost since the 1900s, resulting in today's comparatively limited range of plant-based foods. This alarming loss is the consequence of farmers having been forced to ditch their local varieties for genetically uniform, high-yield crops to keep up with society's demand for 'perfect' food. Think about the way you shop. Do you always grab for those shiny, red, extra-sweet apples, or do you go for the odd-shaped ones with colour imperfections? I was certainly a shiny-red-apple kind of shopper – that was, until I found out that often the types which were exposed to more stressful growing conditions (resulting in imperfections) contain more polyphenols. I now hunt for and celebrate those imperfections. Perhaps the same principle applies to our own life too. Now there's some food for thought.

In terms of our overall diet diversity, it gets worse, with 75 per cent of the world's food being generated from only twelve plant and five animal species. Essentially, this means that both our taste buds and our GM are missing out on so many foods. The consequence? The restricted diet is thought to starve off microbes that require a diverse nutrient supply, and may very well explain why, compared to our ancestors, our GM diversity as a population really has taken quite the hit. I think we can do better, don't you?

> **TAKE-HOME MESSAGE:** *The more diversity in your plant-based diet, the more diverse the nutrient supply for your GM (think dietary fibres, prebiotics and polyphenols). All in all, this equates to a well-fed and diverse range of happy gut microbes, each with their own unique skillset to complement ours.*

So where do you start? It's very much up to you. If you're still working on getting in your minimum daily portion of plant-based foods (two pieces of fruit, five portions of vegetables, three wholegrain portions and one or two portions of nuts, seeds or legumes), don't get overwhelmed by the thought of adding diversity into the mix – stick with the foods you're comfortable with. Once you're feeling confident with your portions, or if you're already ticking that box and want that extra boost, this is where diversity comes into play.

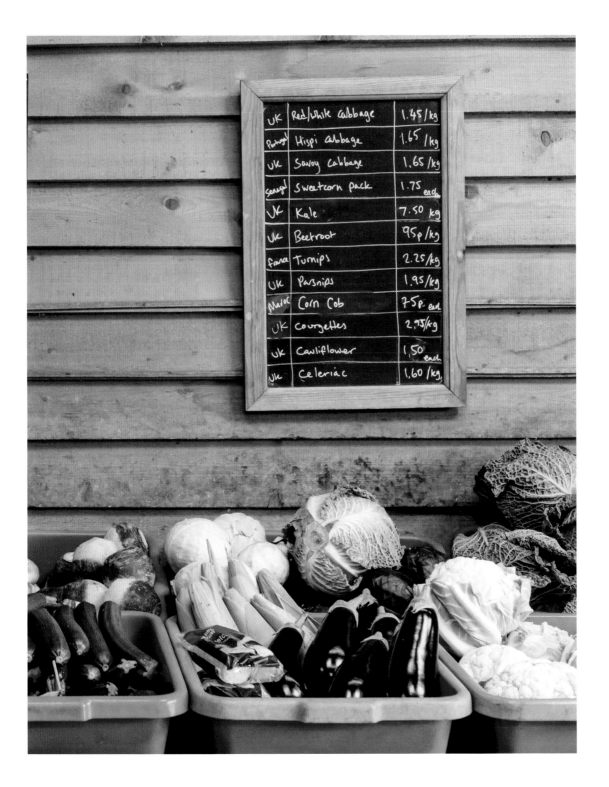

UK	Red/White Cabbage	1.45/kg
Portugal	Hispi Cabbage	1.65/kg
UK	Savoy Cabbage	1.65/kg
Senegal	Sweetcorn pack	1.75 each
UK	Kale	7.50 kg
UK	Beetroot	95p/kg
France	Turnips	2.25/kg
UK	Parsnips	1.95/kg
Maroc	Corn Cob	75p each
UK	Courgettes	2.95/kg
UK	Cauliflower	1.50 each
UK	Celeriac	1.60/kg

Food form

It's not just about what foods we eat, its form also plays a role. I certainly don't want to turn eating into a complex operation that leaves you more exhausted than enthused, but it is worth realizing that the physical structure of a food can affect digestion. For example, my colleagues from King's have demonstrated that, compared to instant oats (the ground oats that turn to porridge in two minutes), the large, coarse oats had a 33 per cent lower effect on blood-sugar levels. This means the sugars were digested more slowly, which is more formally referred to as having a lower glycaemic index, or GI. This suggests that the large, less processed versions are probably better for blood-sugar management, preventing what is commonly referred to as a sugar spike.

What about the health of the environment?

The good news is that prioritizing plant-based foods is much less taxing on the planet too (measured by greenhouse gas emissions). In fact, compared to those who eat a lot of meat, the greenhouse gas emissions for vegetarians are almost 50 per cent lower. If the thought of cutting meat out is a little intimidating, don't worry, I hear you, but cutting down your intake (below 100g/day) still reduces your carbon footprint by over 20 per cent.

Top five switch and saves on your carbon footprint		
THIS ... FOR ... THAT		CARBON-FOOTPRINT SAVING
BEEF (26.5)	legumes (0.5) (see recipe on page 236)	98%
CHEESE (8.5)	cashew cheese (1.5) (see recipe on page 213)	83%
BUTTER (9.5)	avocado (1.5)	86%
CREAM (5.5)	yoghurt (1.5) (see recipe on page 280)	77%
LAMB (25.5)	tofu (1.0) (see recipe on page 226)	96%

Values published in the Journal for Cleaner Production

(Kilograms of greenhouse gases/kilogram of food).

Fasting

To fast or not to fast? Although there is evidence from animal studies that intermittent fasting may benefit our metabolism via its impact on our GM, to date there is little evidence in human studies. There are two main types of intermittent fasting: alternate-day fasting, for example the 5:2 diet, where you consume less than 600 calories on two days and eat normally on the other five days of the week; and time-restricted fasting, for example the 16:8 diet, where you limit your intake to an eight-hour daily eating 'window' and fast the remaining sixteen hours. It is true that these types of diets, when followed, can help with weight management, based on an overall reduction in food intake, simply because you have less opportunity to eat. If you're overweight, losing weight can have many knock-on health benefits. These include lowering blood pressure and blood fats, improving your blood-sugar regulation and lowering your risk of (or even reversing) type 2 diabetes, in some cases. There is also some early-stage evidence that eating in alignment with our body clock has benefits, independent of weight loss. More specifically, increasing our food intake at breakfast (when our body appears to be better primed for food) and reducing it in the evening may improve our body's blood-sugar regulation, even if we don't lose weight. However, as with most diets, they can be difficult to sustain beyond a month or two, and they can impact not only our relationship with food but our mood too (no one enjoys being hungry!). That said, I believe it's very much an individualized approach. It may suit some people, it's just not something I'd recommend to everyone without there being strong evidence behind it. If you are interested in intermittent fasting, why not start by decreasing your current eating window by just an hour either side and see how it feels for you? And if you do want to go the whole way, here are some things to consider: 1. ensure you're still meeting your daily fibre needs (your microbes don't like to starve either); 2. if you have IBS, aim to spread your meals out as much as possible and avoid large meals (as we'll discuss in Chapter 6); and 3. if you take regular medication, check with your GP beforehand as it may affect how they function.

Additional nutrients

This is where things can get a little more complicated. We now know nutrition is certainly not black and white and, no surprise, neither is digestion. I won't bore you with too many details, nor do I want to focus on individual nutrients. It is worth noting, however, that a proportion of nutrients like protein and fat, that escaped digestion in the small intestine, make their way into the large intestine. So it makes sense that they, too, can affect the happiness of our GM, particularly if we over-consume. Like us, our GM is able to digest a wide range of nutrients, so it can survive – well, a core number of microbes, anyway – on pretty much whatever we throw at it. However, there is a vital difference between surviving and thriving. Too many of these nutrients in the large intestine may have some unfavourable side effects. Take protein, for instance. Excess intake can not only result in foul-smelling gas (those who've succumbed to a high-protein diet will know what I mean), but it's also thought to give rise to a more aggressive GM environment, sometimes likened to the concept of 'roid rage'. When our microbes ferment too much protein, they release chemical compounds that have been associated with damaging health outcomes, which have been implicated in colon cancer and inflammatory bowel disease (IBD). More recently, a trial has shown that protein supplementation for ten weeks resulted in a decrease in several health-promoting bacteria, and another study showed a reduction in the beneficial SCFA, butyrate. Further, my and others' research suggests that what may be more important than total protein is the ratio of protein to fibre. This means that if you eat lots of protein (from large portions of foods from animals) but also lots of fibre, the negative impact on your GM is likely reduced. So, if you do enjoy those high-protein animal foods, it's worth siding them with fibre-rich foods including wholegrains, vegetables and legumes, and herbs and spices.

There isn't a great deal of research looking specifically at fat and our microbes. What we do know is that the Mediterranean diet contains around 40 per cent fat and is associated with high GM diversity. Yet other high-fat diets such as the Western diet with a similar ratio of fat are associated with lower GM diversity. This is yet another reason why fixating on individual nutrients is likely unhelpful; it's more about the type of foods you choose. For example, wholegrain sourdough dipped in extra-virgin olive oil is going to be a better option than deep-fried potato wedges dipped in tomato sauce, although the two are equivalent in percentage fat.

What about Omega-3?

Intakes of this type of fat, found in oily fish such as salmon and in plant sources like walnuts and flaxseeds, has been shown to increase SCFA-producing bacteria such as Roseburia. Perhaps the gut–brain axis we touched on in Chapter 2 may also explain, at least in part, the link between omega-3 and improvement in mood disorders. With this in mind, here are five recipes that can help you boost your omega-3 intake.

Five recipes to boost your omega-3 intake

1 QUINOA SUSHI ROLLS, STARRING SMOKED SALMON (PAGE 219)

2 LEMON CURD IN CHIA AND CASHEW TARTLETS (PAGE 257)

3 WALNUT-CENTRED RAW CARROT CAKE BALLS (PAGE 252)

4 SATAY TOFU SKEWERS BEDDED WITH A SIDE OF SAUCY GREENS (PAGE 226)

5 CHEESY VEGAN CRACKERS, SHOWCASING BOTH GROUND AND WHOLE FLAXSEEDS (PAGE 245)

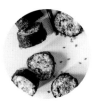   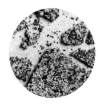

Food additives

Artificial sweeteners are among the most widely used food additives today, including sucralose and aspartame, but is there really such a thing as a free meal? Here's the thing: all additives must undergo a rigorous safety assessment before they're allowed to be included in our food supply. However, historically, the safety assessments haven't considered the impact on our GM – because a lot of these assessments were undertaken before we had a grasp on the importance of it. Some early studies (keeping in mind most are in animals, not humans) demonstrate that certain types of artificial sweeteners (such as sucralose, saccharin and aspartame) negatively impact the GM, promoting blood-sugar issues, liver inflammation and weight gain. Furthermore, a causal relationship (again in animals) has been supported, with studies showing that these negative consequences can be transferred between mice via a poop transplant. At this point, it's worth knowing that only a subset of the results from animal studies actually translate in humans. This is why caution should always be taken when interpreting animal studies. In terms of human studies and artificial sweeteners, the association is not straightforward. There are conflicting findings: some suggest they're beneficial (as an alternative to added sugar), while others suggest they're not so good. These conflicting findings are likely explained by the fact that we all house different microbes which can respond differently. This is illustrated by a very small but important study which showed that daily intake of saccharin at a dose in line with the high end of the 'safe' amount (a level set by health authorities) for one week negatively impacted the blood sugars in only a subset of people. So, when it comes to artificial sweeteners and their impact on your gut microbes, the jury is still out.

Other additives, including a group known as emulsifiers found in a wide range of processed foods, particularly frozen desserts, cakes and biscuits, have also been implicated in triggering pre-diabetes and gut inflammation, at least in mice. My research team are looking to get to the bottom of this with a world-first food-additive trial, to look at the impact of food additives on gut inflammation in people with IBD. I'll be sure to keep you updated.

Salt (more technically known as sodium chloride)

Salt is also added to most processed food. Indeed, around 75 per cent of the salt we eat is already added to processed foods, including breakfast cereals, packet soups, processed meats, snacks such as crisps and biscuits and ready-made meals. Foods containing more than 1.5 grams of salt or 0.6 grams of sodium per 100 grams are considered high in salt. High salt intake can lead to high blood pressure, which is involved in heart disease, and emerging research suggests that our GM may also play an active role in this process. Coincidentally, there have been a number of trials investigating the role of probiotics as a therapy for high blood pressure. Although most have found a small improvement, overall, the size of the benefit means it's probably not worth your money at this point. For now, try the tips below to help reduce your salt intake:

1. CUT THE HABIT:
   Refill your salt shaker on the dinner table with pepper and mixed herbs.

2. TAKE IT SLOWLY:
   Reducing salt gradually over a few months allows your taste buds to adapt and become more sensitive to salt.

3. WATCH PACKET SAUCES:
   Experiment with fresh herbs and spices to bring out the flavours in your dish (see page 59 for inspiration).

Piecing it all together

Okay, so what does the ultimate gut-health diet look like? The truth is, there is no single gut-health diet. There are, however, guiding principles that underpin an eating pattern that supports good gut health. What this looks like in terms of final foods is really up to you, your preferences and where you are on your gut-health journey. This same concept is observed within the 'Blue Zones' – five regions around the world where residents live particularly long and healthy lives. Despite sharing several fundamental principles, including a focus on plant-based foods, many aspects of their diet, including intake of dairy and meat, are inconsistent, with some zones including them and others not. This reinforces the fact that there is no single 'right' way to eat. That said, if you are cutting out entire food groups, you're naturally at an increased risk of a nutritional deficiency. Rest assured: it is possible to get all the nutrients you need from other foods. For instance, in some cultures that limit dairy, they consume calcium-rich bony fish as well as making the most of non-dietary factors that impact bone health, such as getting enough vitamin D from the sun and doing weight-bearing exercises. If the nutritional adequacy of your diet is in doubt, it is best to discuss it with your dietitian or registered nutritionist.

Specific nutrients to consider if you are eating a purely plant-based diet

• Calcium:

Dairy foods are rich in calcium. If you're not eating these, choose calcium-fortified plant-based milks. Other sources include tofu (check on the label that it's set with calcium chloride (E509) or calcium sulphate (E516)), sardines or salmon with bones, and spring greens. Keep in mind that, although spinach contains calcium, it's mostly bound to a compound called oxalate, limiting its absorption.

• Iodine:

Seafood is a good source of iodine. If you don't eat seafood, you may like to consider including sea vegetables in your diet (try the quinoa sushi rolls on page 219). While plant-based foods such as cereals and grains can be a source of iodine, the levels vary depending on the amount of iodine in the soil where the plants were grown.

• Iron:

The iron found in plants (non-haem iron) is less efficiently absorbed. To help your body absorb iron from plant foods, include a source of vitamin C with your meals. Good sources of vitamin C include tomatoes, peppers, oranges and strawberries.

• Omega-3 fats:

Most of the health benefits of omega-3 have been linked to animal-based sources (docosahexaenoic acid, or DHA; and eicosapentaenoic acid, or EPA). Some of the plant-based type of omega-3 (alpha linolenic acid, or ALA) can be converted by our bodies into DHA and EPA. However, the conversion is not efficient, which is why, if you're vegan, it's important to include plenty of the plant-based sources, as discussed on page 65, and consider fortified foods or supplements.

• Selenium:

Meat, fish and nuts are good sources of selenium. If you're purely plant-based, it's best to include nuts in your diet. Brazil nuts top the selenium charts.

• Vitamin B12:

Eggs and dairy are good sources of B12. If vegan consider foods fortified with B12, including fortified plant-based milks and yoghurts. Nutritional yeast is another source, one that I commonly use in cooking for its cheesy flavour profile. Check out my cashew cheese (page 213).

• Zinc:

Phytates found in plant foods such as wholegrains and legumes can reduce zinc absorption. Fermenting (see page 264) and sprouting (see page 267) can help reduce the amount of phytates. Nuts and seeds are also good sources.

Gut health on a plate

As a starting guide, below I have plated an example of what good gut-health eating might look like. This reflects my seven guiding principles opposite that support good gut health. Remember: it's just a guide for you to tweak according to your (and your microbes') preferences.

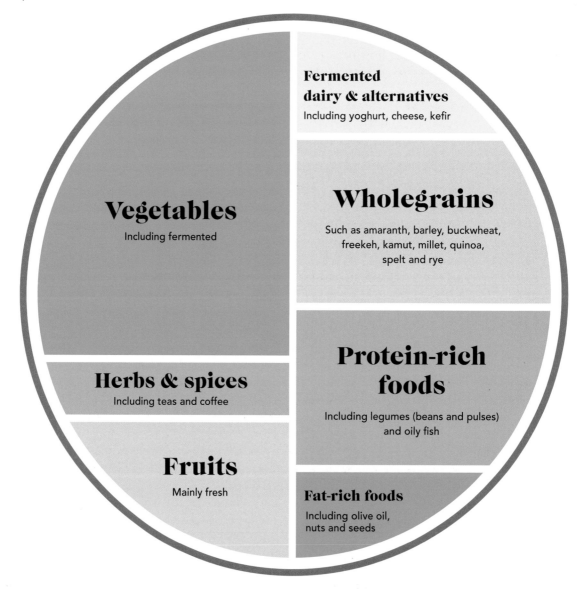

Vegetables
Including fermented

Herbs & spices
Including teas and coffee

Fruits
Mainly fresh

Fermented dairy & alternatives
Including yoghurt, cheese, kefir

Wholegrains
Such as amaranth, barley, buckwheat, freekeh, kamut, millet, quinoa, spelt and rye

Protein-rich foods
Including legumes (beans and pulses) and oily fish

Fat-rich foods
Including olive oil, nuts and seeds

Seven principles

1 **Mostly plants:** From fibre to prebiotics and polyphenols, there is no question that plants are our GM's favourite food.

2 **Diversity all the way:** It's all about feeding and maintaining our diversely skilled team of microbes. Remember: they all prefer different plant-based foods.

3 **Whole and natural versus refined and perfect:** Less waste, more nutrients; it's a no-brainer.

4 **Herb and spice up your life:** There's a whole other world of flavours waiting for your taste buds (and GM) to discover.

5 **Get among legumes (beans and pulses):** The under-rated 'superfood' group loaded with prebiotics and fibre, they're one of the most cost-efficient, nutrient-dense, widely available foods.

6 **Dabble in fermented food:** It really is the ultimate way to engage with our microbial residents, not to mention the incredible flavours and textures that result.

7 **Taste, explore, pause and enjoy:** Food is about more than just our health; it's about community, culture and experiences. Focusing only on the health aspect can sabotage our relationship with food, which, perhaps not surprisingly, is linked with higher rates of gut issues. Our GM can sense the unrest!

Breaking down barriers

When it comes to changing our eating habits, having the knowledge about what to eat is just one hurdle. So let's troubleshoot some of the other common barriers.

Access: Depending on where you live, you may be limited by the range of plant-based foods on offer. My motto is: work with what you've got. TIPS: *1. Modify recipes according to what you have – don't let a few ingredients stop you making a dish; 2. Consider the occasional bulk-buy online, particularly of non-fresh foods such as a diverse range of wholegrains, legumes, nuts, seeds, and so on; 3. Have a go at growing your own fresh herbs, spices and sprouts (see page 267).*

Time: We all have those crazy periods when we tend to push home-made meals way down our priority list. But let me challenge this way of thinking: isn't it exactly during these periods when you need to be on top of your game – can you really afford to get ill when you're so busy? So how do we fit it in? TIPS: *1. Frozen vegetables are underrated; they should be a staple in every busy person's freezer. 2. Cook in bulk for the week ahead or set up a cooking rota with your partner, housemates or work colleagues. 3. Make a list of quick meals; here are some quick options that have saved me on many occasions: the two-minute scram (page 196), thick-protein shake (page 196), and the pistachio and spinach pesto pasta (page 225).*

Cooking: I know the thought of cooking can be intimidating for many. But, from one cooking novice to another, you can't go wrong with most of the recipes in this book. TIPS: *YouTube is a great source for quick and basic cooking tips, like how to boil the perfect egg or use a mandolin slicer.*

Taste: Eating wholesome food can be terribly bland, but so can most foods if you don't dress them right. TIPS: *For me, cooking is all about flaunting a food's assets; often a quick dressing or fifteen minutes in the oven with some olive oil can take a food from a 5/10 to a 10/10.*

Budget: Don't let your diet diversity goals stop you from buying in bulk to save. TIPS: *Team up with a friend and split your purchases or freeze half the portion – most fruit and vegetables last several months in the freezer.*

Plant-based diversity assessment

To get the most out of your diet, a little planning can go a long way. To start off with, it can be helpful to reflect on how many different plant-based foods you're currently eating on a regular basis. Over the past seven days, record the number of different plant-based foods you've eaten.

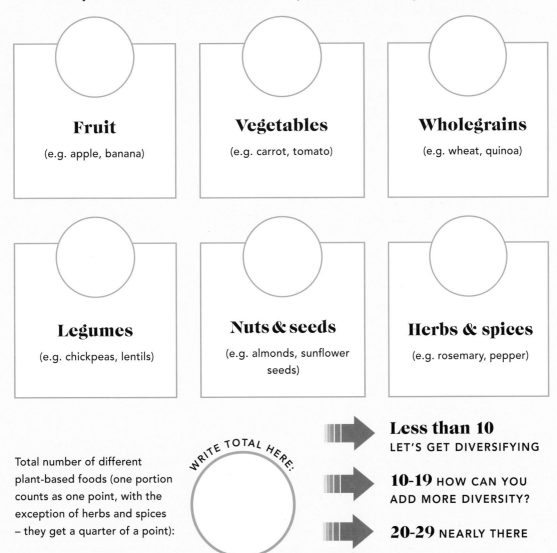

Fruit
(e.g. apple, banana)

Vegetables
(e.g. carrot, tomato)

Wholegrains
(e.g. wheat, quinoa)

Legumes
(e.g. chickpeas, lentils)

Nuts & seeds
(e.g. almonds, sunflower seeds)

Herbs & spices
(e.g. rosemary, pepper)

Total number of different plant-based foods (one portion counts as one point, with the exception of herbs and spices – they get a quarter of a point):

WRITE TOTAL HERE:

Less than 10 LET'S GET DIVERSIFYING

10-19 HOW CAN YOU ADD MORE DIVERSITY?

20-29 NEARLY THERE

30+ WELL DONE!

9 Ways to Diversify Your Diet

(TICK THE STRATEGIES YOU'D LIKE TO TRY)

○ **1** Buy pre-mixed combinations of salad and vegetables (e.g. instead of buying one type of salad leaf, get the one with grated carrot, cabbage and sprouts too).

○ **2** Experiment with grains outside your comfort zone, for example, have you ever tried freekeh? If your local shop doesn't stock it, try online; it travels well.

○ **3** Make a grocery list before you hit the shops to avoid reverting to the same habit buys.

○ **4** Empty a packet of mixed seeds into a glass bottle and leave it on your dining table. It's a great way to remind you to sprinkle them on your meals, as you would pepper.

○ **5** Motivation is a big part of changing habits. If competition gets you going, why not turn this into an office or family challenge?

○ **6** Get the kids involved: allow them to choose, buy and even help prepare and cook their 'new' plant-based food for the week. Taking ownership is a great way to get the family on board.

○ **7** Sometimes, inspiration is half the battle; check out page 59 for a range of plant-based foods worth trying.

○ **8** Mix up your preparation methods. If you steamed your vegetables last night, why not add some olive oil and bake them tonight?

○ **9** Experiment with different combinations of herbs and spices using the tips opposite.

Herb and spice up your life

Keep a range of dried herbs and spices on your kitchen top as a daily reminder.

Start by adding a small amount to your frying pan (two shakes) and taste as you go.

If you're just starting out in the kitchen, opt for the pre-mixed herb and spice combinations, and just start with one per dish.

If you're only adding small amounts and tasting as you go, it's hard to go wrong, but here are some basic combos to build your confidence:

- LEGUMES: Cayenne, chilli, cumin, parsley, sage, thyme

- STIR-FRY: Basil, bay leaves, celery seed, chilli, cinnamon, curry, dill, fennel, garlic, ginger, oregano, parsley, rosemary, smoky paprika, thyme

- SALAD DRESSINGS: Basil, celery seed, chives, dill, fennel, horseradish, mint, mustard, oregano, paprika, parsley, pepper, saffron

- BREADS & CRACKERS: Basil, caraway, cardamom, coriander, cumin, dill, orange peel, oregano, poppy seeds, rosemary, saffron, sage, thyme

- FRUITS: Allspice, anise, cardamom, cinnamon, cloves, coriander, ginger, mint

- DESSERTS: Allspice, anise, cardamom, cinnamon, cloves, fennel, ginger, lemon peel, mace, nutmeg, mint, orange peel, rosemary

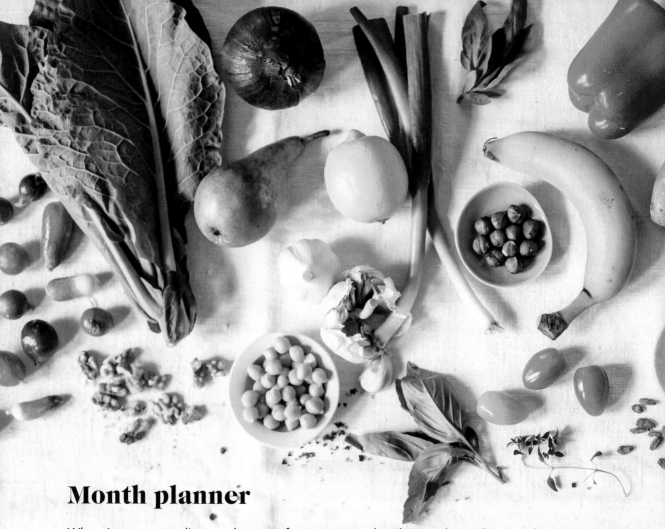

Month planner

When it comes to dietary changes, for most people, slow and steady wins the race. With this in mind, to achieve your diversity target, I find that starting by adding just one or two new varieties each week is the best way to manage and achieve your goal.

WEEK 1: PLANT-BASED FOODS TO TRY	WEEK 2: PLANT-BASED FOODS TO TRY

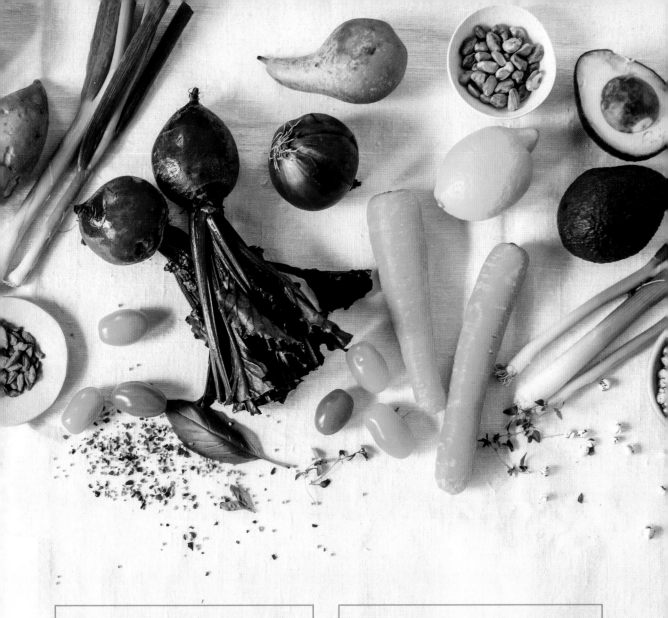

WEEK 3: PLANT-BASED FOODS TO TRY

WEEK 4: PLANT-BASED FOODS TO TRY

CHAPTER 4

Common complaints

Common complaints and how to manage them

Whether it's an occasional inconvenience or a debilitating daily occurrence, no one should have to put up with ongoing gut distress. Unfortunately, many do – in fact, as many as 30 per cent of people worldwide report living with gut symptoms that impact their quality of life. So, what do most do when faced with this type of burden? Check in with Dr Google, of course! Whether it's the convenience factor, the potential for embarrassment or the intimidating thought of a complex array of investigations and medication, many avoid heading straight to their GP – I totally get it.

Instead of turning to the internet, I want to welcome you to this safe, evidence-based space where we'll address the most common gut complaints and discuss practical strategies to help you deal with them. This chapter is certainly not designed to replace your GP or dietitian, but it will point you in the right direction of what you need to do to shake those bothersome symptoms, from simple home solutions to knowing when to visit relevant health-care professionals.

The strategies covered in this chapter are grounded in evidence from good-quality trials, observational studies, expert consensus and sound understanding of how the gut works. Why not just use the top-quality trials? Unfortunately, these trials are not only expensive to undertake but they can't always be done ethically (imagine being in the placebo, fake intervention, group when you know the intervention works). Throughout this chapter, I have of course prioritized the top-quality trials when providing advice. However, where there aren't any, I've suggested strategies, which, although they don't have a wealth of research to back them up, are safe and have worked for many of my patients in clinic. That motto again – let's work with what we've got!

> ✋ **Caution:** If you have a history of disordered eating, please seek support from a dietitian before considering any of the dietary strategies to come. This is because, despite good intentions, focusing on specific aspects of food can trigger negative thoughts and relapse in some.

Before you start testing out the strategies outlined in this chapter it's a good idea to complete the Gut Feelings assessment in Chapter 1 (page 21) so that you have an objective record of your symptoms. For each of the diet strategies, unless otherwise specified, I recommend that you follow the advice for around four weeks. At the end of the four weeks, repeat the same symptom assessment. This will give you an objective idea about whether the intervention worked for you. If there's no improvement, go back to your usual diet and, after a few weeks, reassess your symptoms, then move on to the next strategy. Reassessing the changes in your symptoms once you've returned to your normal diet, although it sounds a bit cumbersome, is actually rather valuable in confirming whether or not it has worked. If your symptoms do improve, this chapter will also look at how to embed the changes into your everyday life without them becoming a burden or placing you at risk of nutritional inadequacies.

Alarm features

It's always best to be on the safe side, so if your gut symptoms are accompanied by any of the below, visit your GP to rule out more troublesome causes:

- *Unintended weight-loss (more than 5 per cent of your body weight in six months)*

- *Blood in your poop*

- *Low blood iron levels*

- *Fever*

- *Family history of cervical or colon cancer, inflammatory bowel disease (IBD) or coeliac disease*

- *New onset of symptoms after 50 years of age*

Assessment: GUT-BRAIN ASSESSMENT

I love this tool, because it helps gauge whether centrally targeted strategies, that is, those which target the messages travelling from your brain to your gut (the gut–brain axis) are going to be important in your management plan. Only complete this if you selected at least three moderate gut symptoms on the Gut Feelings Assessment.

Head over to www.TheGutHealthDoctor.com **to complete the Gut–Brain Assessment and then check back with this book.**

Constipation

The word 'constipation' can mean different things to different people. For some, it's all about how often they poop, whereas others associate it with straining, not emptying their bowels completely or the consistency of their poop. These are all valid descriptions. There are three main subtypes of constipation:

1. **SLOW-TRANSIT CONSTIPATION:** This is when a poop takes a long time to move through the large intestine. This slow movement means there is more time for the water to be absorbed, leaving you with a hard, dry poop.

2. **EVACUATION DISORDER:** Everything moves at a normal speed through the large intestine but something's not quite right with the final 'push', resulting in constipation. This might be due to poorly orchestrated bowel movements involved in pooping, including the intestine, anal trapdoor and pelvic-floor muscles. This means that things are moving, but not in a coordinated fashion (kind of like me on the dance floor). This can result from problematic childhood toileting habits, or be due to physical or structural problems, such as a collapse of the intestinal wall into the vagina (known as a rectocele).

Common symptoms of a rectocele:

- *Feeling like there is something coming down into your vagina – it may feel like you're sitting on a small ball*

- *Feeling or seeing a bulge in or coming out of your vagina*

- *Pressure or pain in your bottom*

- *Discomfort or numbness during sex*

3. **CONSTIPATION-PREDOMINANT IRRITABLE BOWEL SYNDROME (IBS):** There are four types of IBS, and one is dominated by constipation. Although IBS management is discussed in detail in Chapter 6, for some, managing the constipation can improve other symptoms of IBS, including gut pain and bloating. Trying the strategies in this chapter can be a useful first step.

Potential causes of constipation

Low levels of activity	**Stress, anxiety or depression**	**Pregnancy**
Decreased stimulation of gut muscles.	Altered communication via the gut–brain axis.	Both hormonal changes and the physical compression of the uterus on the intestine.
Changes in routine	**Ignoring the urge to go**	**Not eating enough wholegrain fibre**
Our bowels are creatures of habit and changing your eating and sleeping times can confuse them.	This allows more time for the water to be absorbed, resulting in a hard and dry poop, which is difficult for your gut to push out.	Wholegrain fibre can help add bulk to the poop, giving your gut muscles more to work with.
Childhood toileting	**History of physical or psychological abuse**	**Medication or supplements**
Feeling pressured or being regularly interrupted can lead to the development of poor pooping habits.	Trauma can impact the function of muscles involved in pooping via the gut–brain axis.	Different types can impact the bowels, such as directly effecting the gut-muscle movements or increasing fluid absorption.

Taking action

Managing constipation isn't a one-size-fits-all. To help find the strategies that are right for you, I've developed this decision flow diagram. It's as easy as following the arrows and answering the questions as you go. There are three broad areas: diet, physical activity and toilet habits. For best results, try one strategy from each area.

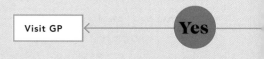

Visit GP ← **Yes**

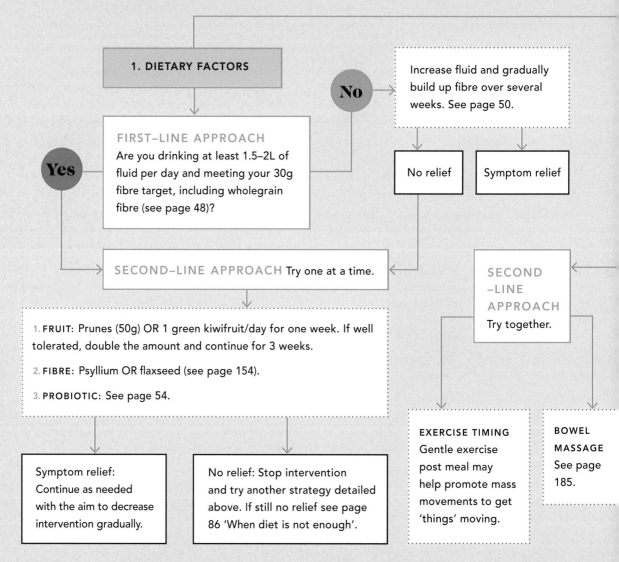

1. DIETARY FACTORS

No → Increase fluid and gradually build up fibre over several weeks. See page 50.

No relief   Symptom relief

FIRST–LINE APPROACH
Are you drinking at least 1.5–2L of fluid per day and meeting your 30g fibre target, including wholegrain fibre (see page 48)?

Yes

SECOND–LINE APPROACH Try one at a time.

SECOND–LINE APPROACH Try together.

1. **FRUIT:** Prunes (50g) OR 1 green kiwifruit/day for one week. If well tolerated, double the amount and continue for 3 weeks.

2. **FIBRE:** Psyllium OR flaxseed (see page 154).

3. **PROBIOTIC:** See page 54.

Symptom relief: Continue as needed with the aim to decrease intervention gradually.

No relief: Stop intervention and try another strategy detailed above. If still no relief see page 86 'When diet is not enough'.

EXERCISE TIMING
Gentle exercise post meal may help promote mass movements to get 'things' moving.

BOWEL MASSAGE
See page 185.

Constipation

DO YOU HAVE ANY ALARM FEATURES?
SEE PAGE 81

No

LIFESTYLE CHANGES

2. PHYSICAL ACTIVITY

3. TOILET HABITS

Yes

FIRST–LINE APPROACH
Do you exercise at least 3 times per week to a level where you'd become short of breath if you tried to sing (for at least 30 minutes)?

No

Whether it's power walking with a friend, going dancing or joining a sports team – regularly moving your body can make a big difference.

ROUTINE
1. Give yourself 5–10 minutes to sit and relax on the toilet; even if you don't poop, make it part of your daily routine. Don't pressure or strain your bowels either, they'll go when they feel comfortable. Some find listening to music or a mindfulness app can help relax them.

2. Aim to sit on the toilet at the same time each day. The mass movement in the morning increases post meal and after coffee, so try to maximize your chances by dedicating time then.

POSITIONING AND TECHNIQUE
1. Check in with your pooping position on page 182.

2. Train your pooping muscles (coordinating the muscles), page 183.

LISTEN TO YOUR BODY
When you get the urge, go! Withholding can cause constipation.

When diet is not enough . . .

Like each of us, our bowels are unique and have their own 'personality'. Some are laid-back and easy-going, while others can be a little more uptight and reliant on routine. This explains why there is no one strategy or medication that suits all. Take two of my patients: thirty-nine-year-old Sally and twenty-seven-year-old Jenny. They both presented with near-identical gut symptoms but, as I got to know more about each of them, it became strikingly clear how different their bowel personalities were. Sally's bowels were a happy-go-lucky type which just needed more fibre to give the muscles something to work with. Psyllium worked a treat, followed by increasing wholegrains in her diet, for long-term maintenance. Then there was Jenny. At face value, it seemed Jenny's bowels were plain old stubborn. Jenny had a high-fibre diet, drank plenty of water and exercised five days a week. When she came to me she was juggling different laxatives, struggling to get the balance right in terms of dose and frequency, having had many 'close calls' at work. We sat together and got to know Jenny's bowels. We learned that they were not stubborn but shy: they didn't like opening anywhere but in the comfort of her own home. In fact, when Jenny was housesitting with her boyfriend, her bowels were so self-conscious they didn't open all week. For Jenny's bowels, it was all about creating a feeling of comfort and safety. We started off by establishing a relaxing morning bowel routine, while slowly cutting down the laxatives. Jenny also started using the poop-pourri (see recipe opposite) when she needed to go outside of her comfort zone. Within three weeks Jenny was laxative-free and not only had her bowel confidence been boosted, her anxiety had reduced, with no more worrying about laxative-related incidents.

Laxatives

In cases where things are pretty 'backed up', sometimes you need an extra push to get things moving, at least initially. It's always best to discuss with your pharmacist before starting, as some laxatives could make some conditions worse. There are also laxatives that your GP can prescribe if over-the-counter laxatives are not effective. If you find yourself depending on laxatives for more than a week, visit your GP to discuss different options.

Poop-pourri

Now, don't laugh: this really will revolutionize your bathroom experience. Not only does it smell so much more natural and subtle than traditional toilet sprays, it's a tenth of the price, and so much more efficient at getting the 'job' done too. You see, the role of this concoction is not to mask the smell in the air that escapes the toilet bowl but rather to trap the smell inside the toilet bowl. Now, I know it sounds a little too good to be true, but it's no marketing scam, it's just based on simple science! Unlike traditional sprays, with this, you spray it directly into the bowl before you go. The oily mix forms a thin film across the water in the toilet, so when you go it traps the smell under the film (which is just a mix of gases produced by our GM). When you flush the toilet, the smell is gone – like magic. It also makes a very memorable (and affordable) present for your friends and family.

**You will need a 60ml glass spray bottle
(plastic is okay for short-term use)**

INGREDIENTS:

essential oils of choice (I like peppermint and a combo of lavender and vanilla)

1 tbsp rubbing alcohol (this is super-cheap online, or you can use 2 tbsp vodka)

1 pea-size drop of body wash or washing-up liquid (helps combine the oil and water)

distilled water (tap water is fine if you use within one month)

METHOD:

1. Place 10–15 drops of the essential oils and alcohol in your spray bottle and shake well.

2. Add the body wash or washing-up liquid and fill the bottle up to the neck with water. Shake well.

3. Place in your bathroom with written instructions for any guests to shake before spraying four squirts into the toilet bowl, pre-poop.

Bloating

Bloating is one of the most common gut symptoms people report and can be rather distressing, especially when the cause is unexplained.

Simply speaking, bloating is the feeling of increased pressure in your intestine that may be accompanied by visible protrusion (aka 'food baby'). The causes and mechanics of bloating are complex. The built-up pressure can result from the sheer volume of food or fluid you've eaten or from gas produced by our gut microbiota (GM) when it's fed large amounts of fermentable carbohydrates, including some types of fibre. This increase in gut content essentially stretches the intestine, giving you the sensation of bloating. But why do some people experience bloating and others don't, even when they eat and drink the same type and amount of food? There are many reasons, but one of the most common is the sensitivity of your intestine. A heightened sensitivity, known as visceral hypersensitivity, is particularly common in people with functional gut disorders like IBS. Visceral hypersensitivity has been demonstrated in studies that use MRI (special scans that can measure gas inside your intestines). What they have shown is that, despite the same amount of gas being present, people with IBS, or other functional gut disorders, are more likely to feel bloated than those without them.

Susceptibility to bloating can also depend on the balance between how much gas your unique GM produces and how efficient your body is at absorbing it. The transport of gas through the intestine can also be an issue for some, resulting in trapped gas. Many of the strategies discussed below, such as gentle stretching, abdominal massage and heat packs, can help release trapped gas.

In a subset of people with functional gut disorders, bloating can also be exaggerated by an inappropriate movement of the diaphragm (the dome-shaped sheet of muscle that helps us breathe) and the belly. This results in belly protrusion, which people frequently describe as making them look several months pregnant, even though they're not. It's similar to when you take a big breath into your belly, pushing it out, except it happens unconsciously. Unlike standard bloating, this has nothing to do with what's in your intestine per se; instead, it's considered a reflex related to tummy pain or discomfort whereby the gut triggers the brain via the gut–brain axis and, in an attempt to relieve the gut distress, the brain contracts the diaphragm and relaxes the tummy muscles. The fix? Once the trigger of the tummy pain or discomfort is managed (whether it is IBS, constipation or another cause), the belly protrusion also typically resolves. In my clinic I've also found that spending five minutes doing some

What are 'functional' gut disorders?

It's a category of conditions that include IBS where the structure of the gut is normal but the function isn't. Somewhat like a show house or a model home, everything looks okay but, on closer inspection, often the plumbing and electricity don't actually work. If it turns out that this applies to your gut, don't panic, as such disorders really are very common, something we'll assess on page 139.

diaphragmatic breathing each day for at least eight weeks can help you become more aware of when this reflex is triggered; in turn, this can help you to consciously release the over-contracted diaphragm (see page 173).

There are two main types of bloating, continuous and intermittent. Continuous bloating is always present, with no daily fluctuations or association with what you eat. This type could be related to the reflex discussed above but may also be a sign that something more troublesome is going on, so it's best to visit your GP to be on the safe side. Intermittent bloating is more common, and often people report their symptoms are worse towards the end of the day or after a meal. This type is most often managed through diet and lifestyle strategies.

It's important to be aware that occasional bloating is normal, particularly if we've had a heavy meal or eaten extra fibre. In fact, a bit of bloating after a high-fibre meal is a good thing. It's a sign of a well-fed GM that's doing its job.

Despite the complexity of the causes of bloating, in many cases it can be reduced, or even eliminated, with simple changes to diet and lifestyle. These self-management strategies can be broken down into two stages in order of difficulty, starting with low-burden strategies and working up. As always, it's up to you which stage you start at, but I recommend starting with the 'low-hanging fruit', so to speak, and working through the more time-consuming strategies only if needed. For many people, first-line strategies are enough.

1. First-line strategies

Diet:

- **AVOID LARGE MEALS.** Split food intake into smaller portions, eating four or five meals spread across the day.

- **TAKE TIME TO CHEW YOUR FOOD WELL,** aiming for between ten and twenty chews per mouthful. It can also help to get into the habit of putting down your knife and fork after each mouthful to remind yourself to take time to chew.

- Although the evidence is limited, **AVOID SWALLOWING EXCESS AIR** from carbonated drinks, drinking through a straw and chewing gum.

- **AVOID ADDED POLYOLS** that are commonly found in sugar-free foods and chewing gum, such as mannitol, maltitol, sorbitol, xylitol and isomalt.

- **ARE YOU OVERDOING IT ON FERMENTED FOODS** (e.g. kefir, sauerkraut)? Halve your portions for two weeks and reassess. If your symptoms improve, continue with smaller portions and look to gradually increase over time, if appropriate.

- **KEEP TO NO MORE THAN ONE PIECE OF FRUIT PER SITTING** (approx. 80g fresh, 30g dried), with up to three per day.

- **AVOID SMOOTHIES AND JUICES.** Opt for whole foods instead.

Lifestyle:

- **AVOID WEARING TIGHT CLOTHES.** I know this sounds a little odd, but 'tight pants syndrome' is actually a thing! It was first described in a medical journal back in 1993.

- **GENTLE EXERCISE AND STRETCHING CAN HELP DIFFUSE TRAPPED GAS.** Check out the yoga flow on page 172.

- **BETTER OUT THAN IN.** Go for a walk outside and 'deflate'.

- **TRY PEPPERMINT-OIL CAPSULES.** Peppermint oil has been shown to relax your gut muscles and therefore may help relieve bloating triggered by trapped gas. The evidence for peppermint oil and bloating is based on people with IBS. See page 155.

- **TRY USING A HEAT PACK.** Placing a heat pack (or a damp towel that's been warmed) on your belly can help loosen up the gut muscles, which may relieve trapped gas. It also recruits more blood flow to the area, which may settle overactive gut muscles.

It's up to you whether you want to try one strategy at a time or choose a few. If symptoms do improve with multiple strategies, you may like to reintroduce each strategy one by one. This will help you to assess which are most beneficial so you're not burdened with too many changes in the long term. If you don't get symptom relief from the first-line strategies, move on to the second-line strategies.

Remember: Include chosen strategies in your gut health action plan on page 282.

2. Second-line strategies

Diet:

- **CHECK FOR FOOD INTOLERANCES** – see Chapter 5.

- **HALVE YOUR PORTIONS OF KEY HIGHER-FODMAP FOODS** from the table on page 151 for two weeks. If symptoms improve, reintroduce as per STAGE 2: REINTRODUCTION on page 152. If symptoms only slightly improve you may like to consider the full FODMAP-lite approach on pages 152–153.

Additional therapies:

- **CONSIDER STRATEGIES THAT TARGET THE GUT–BRAIN AXIS** in Chapter 7.

- **DISCUSS FURTHER INVESTIGATIONS WITH YOUR GP**, including small intestinal bacterial overgrowth (SIBO) (page 156) and coeliac disease (page 111).

Bloating can also be a side effect of constipation and diarrhoea. If you suffer with either, make sure you check out those symptom-specific strategies too (pages 84–85 and 96).

Although we tend to blame bloating all on diet, I find this is rarely the case. This was certainly true for one of my patients, twenty-nine-year-old Catherine. Catherine was an ex-gymnast who, although professionally retired, was still training most days. She struggled with bloating, alongside what she called 'moody bowels' for several years (the type that switch from hard to loose from one week to the next). But it wasn't until she was out at a dinner party and received the attempted compliment, 'You look fantastic, how far along are you?' that Catherine was driven to take action. In my clinic, Catherine told me the details of her diet and lifestyle and opened up about her history of anorexia. Although she had recovered from her eating disorder, it was apparent that her bowels were still in the process of repairing themselves. I explained to Catherine that, just like our arm and leg muscles, we can also lose gut muscle when severely malnourished, as in the case of anorexia. As a result, the way in which the nerves and gut muscles communicate can become impaired, resulting in these bothersome gut symptoms. I also reinforced the message that, although, for most, this nerve–muscle communication tends to resolve with time, it was important to be realistic with her expectations and to acknowledge that things can take a little longer for some than it might for others. Catherine had also recognized that the more frustrated she got with her bloating, the worse it seemed to get.

How did we approach it? Slowly and gently was the key. We identified several lifestyle factors, including stress (particularly food-related fears from previous learned behaviours) and wearing tight gym gear all day. In terms of diet, Catherine was taking large amounts of a prebiotic supplement (which she had read was good for her gut), so we cut that out and focused on getting all her required nutrition from five smaller meals spread across the day. We didn't restrict any foods but instead broadened her diet in line with the gut health on a plate principles from Chapter 3. Over the following six months Catherine managed to get on top of her gut symptoms and also noticed an improvement in her mental health. In fact, when I asked her how she was feeling, she remarked, after a moment of thought, 'You know what, I feel like a new woman.'

Diarrhoea

Loose or watery poop occurs when there is either too much fluid secreted into the intestine or not enough fluid reabsorbed into your body. Here is a fun fact for you. On average, a massive nine litres of fluid enters the small intestine each day, mainly from body secretions, of which 90 per cent is normally reabsorbed.

When thinking about how to manage diarrhoea, you need to consider whether it's an acute (short-term) or chronic (longer-term) issue. Diarrhoea can also come with other symptoms, such as urgency (not being able to hold it back). If you're nodding right now, rest assured, there are several strategies to help you get on top of it, particularly the chronic type, which is something no one should have to live with.

Acute diarrhoea

Acute diarrhoea is often caused by the invasion of unfriendly microbes into the intestine. This may last from a few days to several weeks, and includes traveller's diarrhoea, viral gastroenteritis ('enteritis' meaning inflammation of the small intestine) and food poisoning. This type of diarrhoea can also occur when you start on a new medication, including antibiotics. Acute diarrhoea is best managed by your GP, who can assess whether medication is needed.

- **TRAVELLER'S DIARRHOEA** This is the most common illness in travellers visiting developing countries, with reports suggesting that it affects between 20 and 50 per cent of travellers. Although the diarrhoea is usually mild and can be self-managed, as many as 10 per cent of sufferers may go on to subsequently develop what is called post-infectious IBS (discussed in Chapter 6). It's best to see your GP before taking any anti-diarrhoeal medication for acute diarrhoea, as it may prolong an infection, trapping the culprit in the intestine.

- **ANTIBIOTIC-ASSOCIATED DIARRHOEA (AAD)** Although antibiotics are crucial in fighting off some bacterial infections, they can also disrupt your GM, which can result in diarrhoea. As many as 30 per cent of people are said to experience loose poops when taking antibiotics. To combat this, taking a specific probiotic during your antibiotic therapy, and continuing for a week post-antibiotics has been shown to significantly decrease your risk of AAD.

Chronic diarrhoea

Chronic diarrhoea is a non-specific symptom that can occur because of a functional gut disorder or be due to a more sinister problem. If it's accompanied by any of the alarm features on page 81, visit your GP as a first step.

Treatment of chronic diarrhoea is best achieved by managing the underlying cause. This might mean identifying a food intolerance or identifying and medically managing the disease (e.g. IBD). There are also several strategies that can help manage symptoms, particularly if symptoms persist following medical management.

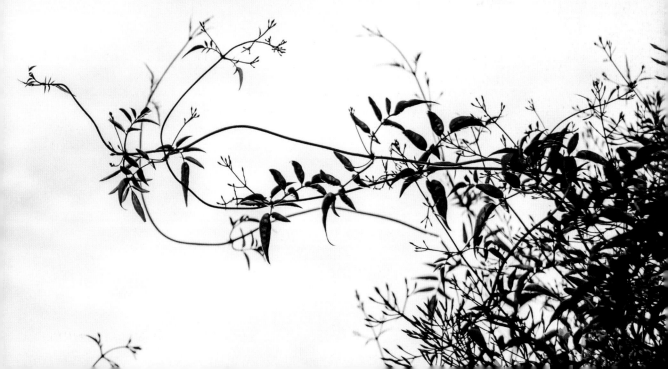

Diet strategies:

- **EAT SMALLER, MORE FREQUENT MEALS** – a good rule of thumb is to divide your current meals into five or six smaller meals across the day, meaning you don't change the total amount you eat, just your eating pattern.

- **LIMIT FOODS AND FLUIDS THAT MAY STIMULATE THE COLON,** such as chilli, high-fat meals, coffee and alcohol.

- **LIMIT KEY SOURCES OF FERMENTABLE CARBOHYDRATES** (higher-FODMAP foods; see page 151) for two weeks, followed by reintroduction (page 152).

- **IF DIARRHOEA IS SEVERE, ENSURE ADEQUATE HYDRATION** with electrolyte solution, such as Dioralyte. This is needed when fluid is passing 'straight through'.

- **CONSIDER PSYLLIUM HUSK** This is a water-loving fibre that can help thicken your poop output. Check out page 154 for details.

Lifestyle strategies:

- **AVOID NICOTINE,** which may stimulate gut movements.

- If suffering with urgency or pooping mishaps, **DAILY PELVIC FLOOR EXERCISES** can help (see page 184).

- If psyllium does not help, **DISCUSS THE USE OF AN ANTI-DIARRHOEAL WITH YOUR GP**. This will slow down gut movement, allowing more time for gut fluid to be reabsorbed. First-line anti-motility medications include loperamide.

NOTE: *Anti-motility medications may be less well tolerated in diarrhoea-predominant IBS.*

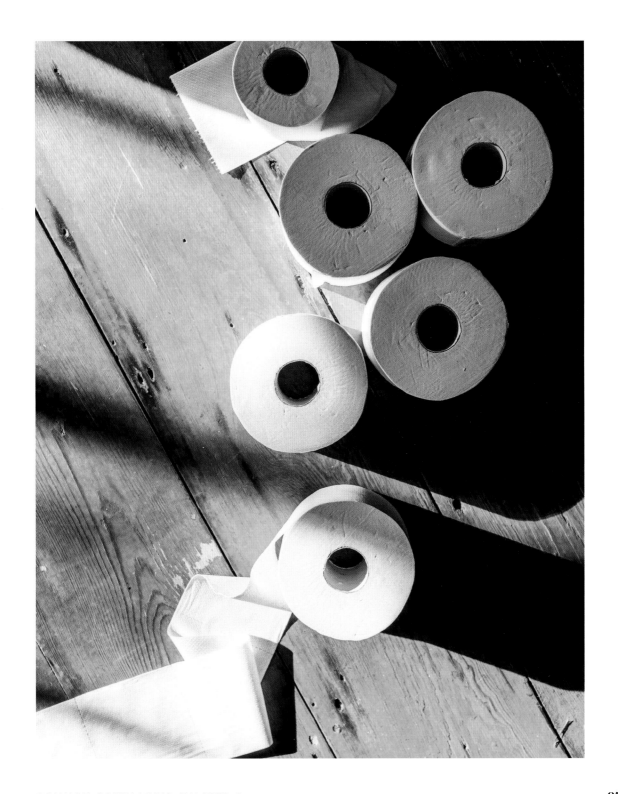

Flatulence

Breaking wind, blowing a raspberry, letting one rip – however you refer to it, flatulence is a normal, healthy phenomenon. The average person meeting their daily 30 grams of fibre passes flatus (wind) between ten and twenty times a day. This is a sign of a well-fed GM, but if flatulence becomes persistently excessive or the smell is a cause for a building evacuation and it interferes with your work or social life, it's worth reading on.

Gas in our intestines comes from two main sources, from the air we breathe in and as the by-product of GM fermentation in the large intestine, that is, from our GM digesting our food leftovers. When it comes to flatulence, it's the gas produced by our GM that is the most relevant source. This explains why around 70 per cent of total gas in the intestine in healthy people is found in the large intestine.

When looking to manage flatulence, as daft as it may sound, it's worth considering which aspect bothers you. Typically, if you're passing wind less than twenty times a day, it's more likely other factors that are bothering you. Think: is it the odour, the inability to hold it back or the soiling of underwear that can sometimes occur? Although each can be socially embarrassing, if you identify the problem, it will help inform the most effective management strategies to solve it.

Excess gas

Excess gas is typically the result of excess GM fermentation, which may mean that you've overfed your GM. There are many causes for excess GM fermentation:

- **EXCESS FOOD RESIDUE:** Our GM engages in a feeding frenzy if too much food gets to the large intestine. This can occur in several scenarios, for example when food travels too fast through the small intestine (diarrhoea); if you're unable to digest specific food components (food intolerance); or if you have a really high-fibre diet or rapidly increase the amount of fibre in your diet.

- **CONSTIPATION:** If things travel extra slowly through the large intestine, the GM gets more time to ferment the leftover food bits that would otherwise have exited into the toilet bowl.

- **SIBO:** When a considerable number of bacteria travel up from the large intestine into the small intestine (SIBO), these bacteria suddenly have access to all that lovely food which they didn't have access to in the large intestine (see page 156 for more on SIBO).

Odour

Interestingly, more than 99 per cent of the gas produced by our GM, including hydrogen, methane and carbon dioxide, is odourless. So where's the smell coming from? That distinct whiff of rotten egg is caused by bacteria breaking down sulphur-containing compounds in our diet. This produces trace amounts of sulphur-containing gases such as hydrogen sulphide. Food and/or drinks high in sulphur-containing compounds include those high in specific amino acids (the building blocks of protein: cysteine, methionine and taurine). These include protein supplements, meat, chicken, eggs, and so on. Sulphur-containing compounds are also found in cruciferous vegetables (e.g. broccoli, cauliflower, cabbage, kale, Brussels sprouts, turnips), allium vegetables (e.g. garlic, onion, leeks, chives) and additives (e.g. some beer and wine). Now, before you go cutting out these types of vegetables, it's worth noting that many of their sulphur-containing compounds are known to have a range of health benefits, and their rotten-egg potential is also much lower than high-protein foods such as protein supplements (both whey- and plant-based). Therefore, targeting the excess-protein intake is a better place to start. Interestingly, in contrast to traditional thinking, research from Dr Yao and colleagues suggests that increasing fibre, rather than restricting it, may in fact help manage pungent flatulence. How? By increasing the availability of dietary fibre, our GM is kept busy feeding on that and is less likely to ferment the sulphur-containing amino acids found in high-protein foods.

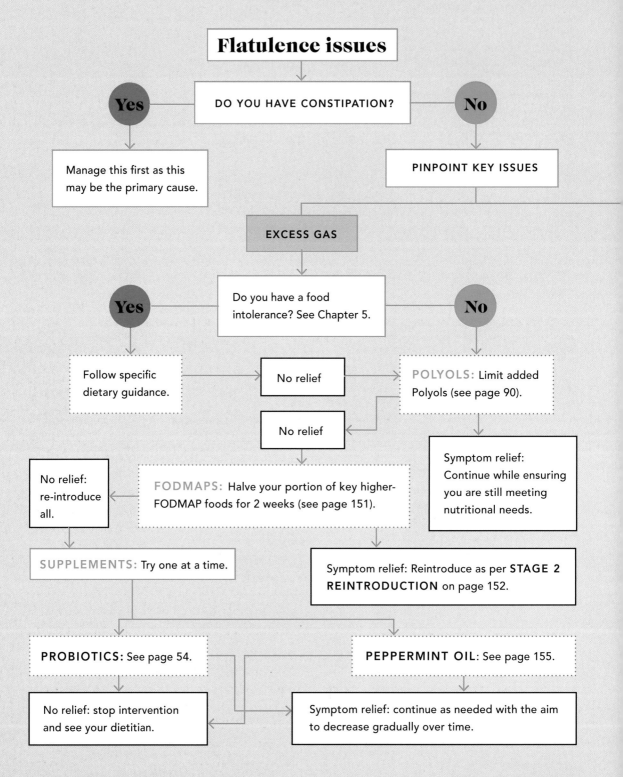

Flatulence issues

Yes ← **DO YOU HAVE CONSTIPATION?** → **No**

Manage this first as this may be the primary cause.

PINPOINT KEY ISSUES

EXCESS GAS

Yes ← Do you have a food intolerance? See Chapter 5. → **No**

Follow specific dietary guidance. → No relief → **POLYOLS:** Limit added Polyols (see page 90).

No relief

FODMAPS: Halve your portion of key higher-FODMAP foods for 2 weeks (see page 151).

No relief: re-introduce all.

Symptom relief: Continue while ensuring you are still meeting nutritional needs.

SUPPLEMENTS: Try one at a time.

Symptom relief: Reintroduce as per **STAGE 2 REINTRODUCTION** on page 152.

PROBIOTICS: See page 54.

PEPPERMINT OIL: See page 155.

No relief: stop intervention and see your dietitian.

Symptom relief: continue as needed with the aim to decrease gradually over time.

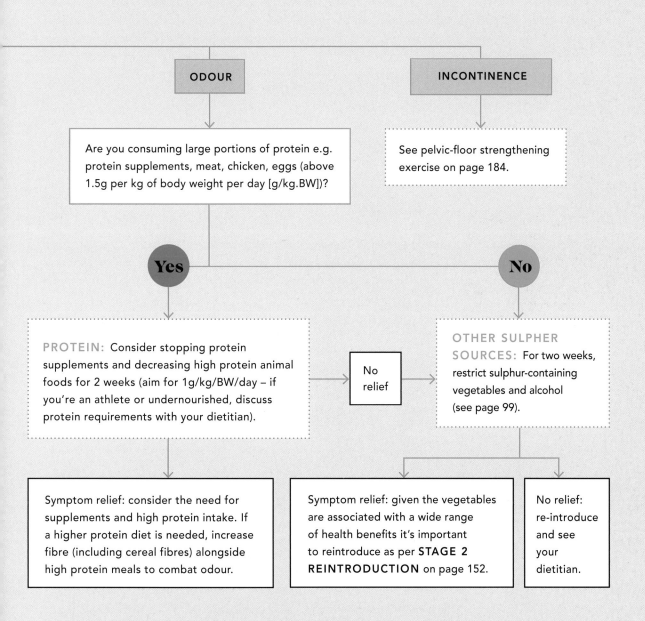

ODOUR

INCONTINENCE

Are you consuming large portions of protein e.g. protein supplements, meat, chicken, eggs (above 1.5g per kg of body weight per day [g/kg.BW])?

See pelvic-floor strengthening exercise on page 184.

Yes

No

PROTEIN: Consider stopping protein supplements and decreasing high protein animal foods for 2 weeks (aim for 1g/kg/BW/day – if you're an athlete or undernourished, discuss protein requirements with your dietitian).

No relief

OTHER SULPHER SOURCES: For two weeks, restrict sulphur-containing vegetables and alcohol (see page 99).

Symptom relief: consider the need for supplements and high protein intake. If a higher protein diet is needed, increase fibre (including cereal fibres) alongside high protein meals to combat odour.

Symptom relief: given the vegetables are associated with a wide range of health benefits it's important to reintroduce as per **STAGE 2 REINTRODUCTION** on page 152.

No relief: re-introduce and see your dietitian.

Heartburn and acid reflux

Despite its misleading name and the location of the symptoms, heartburn has nothing to do with the heart but is all about your oesophagus (food pipe). Heartburn is a common symptom of reflux, where acid travels in the wrong direction, up from your stomach and into your oesophagus via the trapdoor (i.e. the oesophageal sphincter we covered in Chapter 1). Unlike your stomach, your oesophagus isn't built for harsh acid and, as a result, it triggers a nasty burning sensation in the chest – heartburn.

Most people will experience heartburn if they overfill their stomach (think Christmas dinner) and thus create an unequal pressure between the stomach and oesophagus. When this pressure imbalance reaches a certain level, it essentially lifts the trapdoor and allows acid to flow upwards into the oesophagus. If, however, you're experiencing heartburn and/or reflux regularly (at least twice a week) and it's not related to overeating, you may have what is called gastro-oesophageal reflux disease (GORD). GORD is a common condition, affecting as many as 10 per cent of adults. Although some people are genetically more susceptible to reflux, and others have a physical cause such as a hiatus hernia, there are several key diet and lifestyle factors (outlined overleaf) that can decrease your risk of GORD.

Not all heartburn occurs because of acid reflux. This more recent discovery explains why, for some people, acid reflux medications (even the strong ones) provide no relief. This type of heartburn, where there is no clinical explanation or abnormal test, is termed 'functional heartburn' (yes, that 'functional' word again). Like the other functional gut disorders, a sensitive intestine, related to the dysfunction between the gut and the brain, is thought to play a role.

This was the case with one of my patients, fifty-two-year-old Tom. Tom had been bothered by symptoms of heartburn on and off for ten years, although, over the last year, his symptoms had become progressively worse. Tom's GP had prescribed him a proton pump inhibitor (which works to lower stomach-acid production). After several months and no benefit (despite increasing the dose), he was referred for an endoscopy (where they pass a camera down the oesophagus) to take a look at what was going on. He also had other tests to find out how the oesophagus was moving and how much acid was entering. All the tests came back normal. At this stage, Tom was at a bit of a loss as to what was going on, so decided to come and see me. He explained that he had tried all the standard diet strategies, but none of them had worked. Appreciating the functional nature of Tom's symptoms, we went into detail not only about Tom's diet but also other lifestyle factors, including sleep, stress, hobbies, and so on. He also opened up about his recent marriage breakdown, which was causing him a lot of stress.

We decided not to change Tom's diet (he felt this stressed him out more) and started with some basic daily mindfulness and sleep strategies (see Chapter 7). I reinforced to Tom that to see the benefit he had to really commit to these daily strategies. To help with this we went through a number of habit-forming tips (see page 288). Eight weeks later Tom returned, his stress down and his quality of sleep up. The severity of his heartburn had also eased off, although he was still feeling it most days. Having experienced some benefit, Tom was keen to take the next step and readdress some of those diet strategies, including reducing his alcohol intake and the size of his evening meal – both of which he'd previously tried, with only limited success. Four weeks after that Tom emailed me to express his gratitude and to say that he didn't need another appointment, as he had his symptoms under control.

So, what is the evidence behind diet and lifestyle strategies for managing heartburn and reflux? I'll be frank with you: it is minimal in terms of good-quality trials. But there are observational studies, and consensus from leading experts, which support trying these strategies before opting for medication. If there is a part of you that's tempted to skip these strategies and just go straight for the meds – because, let's face it, they can be easier to implement – keep in mind that some reflux medications may impact your GM. Of course, if you need medication, you need it – it's all about weighing up the pros and cons. For those tempted to just put up with the symptoms, it's important to be aware that chronic reflux is not only burdensome for you in terms of the discomfort but can also increase your risk of diseases such as oesophageal cancer – so whichever pathway you decide to take, getting on top of it is really important.

Diet strategies – short term:

- **AVOID LARGE MEALS.** Split food intake into smaller portions, eating five or six meals across the day.

- **ALLOW AT LEAST THREE HOURS** between your last meal of the day and bedtime.

- **COMPLETE A SEVEN-DAY FOOD AND SYMPTOM DIARY** (using My Gut Diary; see page 124) and look for any patterns between foods, lifestyle factors and your symptoms. Although evidence is limited, commonly reported diet triggers include high-fat meals, e.g. deep-fried foods and pastries (switch to the grilled and wholegrain options), carbonated beverages, citrus fruits/juices (try herbal teas such as ginger instead), tomatoes, spicy foods (switch to another flavoursome herb, like smoky paprika or turmeric), chocolate, caffeine (opt for decaffeinated drinks) and alcohol.

Diet strategies – long term:

- **KEEP YOUR WEIGHT IN CHECK,** as being overweight is linked with a higher risk of reflux. This is because the extra weight increases the pressure placed on your oesophageal sphincter.

- **CONSTIPATION AND BLOATING MAY ALSO WORSEN REFLUX** – ensure these are well managed.

Alarm Features

If you have any of the red flags below, don't hold off. Discuss with your GP straight away:
- **DIFFICULTY SWALLOWING**
- **ANY LUMPS OR TENDERNESS IN YOUR THROAT OR BELLY**
- **FAMILY HISTORY OF EITHER OESOPHAGEAL OR STOMACH CANCER**

Lifestyle strategies:

- **DE-STRESS WITH BREATHING EXERCISES** (see page 173). It all comes back to the gut–brain axis, where mental stress can trigger physical stress along your intestine.

- **AVOID TIGHT CLOTHING**, like high-waisted jeans or a tight bra.

- **STOP SMOKING.** I know it's easier said than done. Nicotine, the key part of tobacco, is thought to relax the oesophageal sphincter, which means acid can move up in the wrong direction, leading to reflux and heartburn.

- **IF YOU GET REFLUX WHILE IN BED OR SLEEPING**, try lying on your left-hand side. Why? The oesophagus is connected to the right side of the stomach, which means that lying on the left prevents the acid from being pushed back up the oesophagus.

- **RAISE ONE END OF YOUR BED** by ten to twenty centimetres so that both your head and your chest are at a level just above your waist.

Other strategies for acid reflux:

- **NON-STEROIDAL ANTI-INFLAMMATORY DRUGS** may make symptoms worse. The most common types include ibuprofen, aspirin, naproxen and diclofenac. If you're unsure, check with your pharmacist.

- **CHAT TO YOUR PHARMACIST** about different types of over-the-counter medication. The most common include antacids, which help to neutralize the acid (available as a liquid or a chewable tablet, like Rennie). Some antacids are also combined with alginates (e.g. Gaviscon); this forms a foam layer on top of your stomach contents, preventing the acid from moving back up the oesophagus. There are also histamine H2-receptor antagonists (such as ranitidine) and proton-pump inhibitors (such as omeprazole), which decrease the production of stomach acid. If you're relying on over-the-counter medications at least twice a week for long periods, it's worth a visit to your GP.

Exercise-associated gut discomfort

Despite the many benefits of exercise, strenuous endurance activities can cause gut discomfort in many people. This can not only impact on our enjoyment of exercise but also on our ability to refuel whilst doing it, leading to impaired performance and delayed recovery. If you are currently struggling with exercise-associated gut discomfort, here are some strategies worth trying. Remember: Every gut is different, so do what works for you.

1. **HYDRATION:** Ensure you are well hydrated before starting exercise (which means paying attention to your thirst both the day before and on the day) and continue to hydrate during exercise where possible. How much exactly? It's difficult to put a figure on how much you need to drink; instead, current recommendations suggest a 'drink to thirst' approach is the best way to maintain optimal hydration around exercise. For exercise lasting under two hours, water will suffice but, for longer events, a standard sports drink which contains electrolytes might be better tolerated.

2. **PRE-EVENT DIET:** If you have experienced exercise-associated gut discomfort before, try restricting the key higher-FODMAP foods (see table on page 151) from your diet between twenty-four and forty-eight hours prior to strenuous endurance training and/or events. There is growing evidence to suggest that restricting these foods (or a more formal low-FODMAP diet, as discussed on page 147) before an event may benefit those prone to exercise-associated gut discomfort, reducing symptoms both during and after exercise. That said, reintroducing these foods after the event is important to support good overall gut health. Visit a registered sports dietitian for individualized support.

3. **PRE-EXERCISE MEAL:** Everyone's digestion is different, but having your last main meal between two and four hours before strenuous endurance training and/or an event is likely to decrease gut discomfort. If you do have a snack closer to the exercise, opt for foods lower in fibre, protein and fat because these will be more rapidly digested (decreasing the potential for gut discomfort when starting the exercise). My go-to snack is a crumpet with jam and half a ripe banana.

4. **DURING EXERCISE:** Training the gut to tolerate feeding during exercise is an important part of training for endurance events lasting longer than two hours. Why two hours? This is, on average, how long our body's energy stores can sustain

exercise of at least a moderate intensity. It's best to incorporate nutrition training into your event-training programme to increase gut tolerance and reduce the risk of symptoms. High-carbohydrate, low-fibre options are best for eating during exercise.

If you are struggling with underlying gut symptoms and are new to exercise, start with lower-impact exercise, such as power walking, cycling, cross-training machines or swimming and build up the duration and intensity over several months.

As we come to the end of what I consider the 'bread and butter' of gut complaints, I hope you're feeling more informed and confident to tackle those bothersome symptoms as they arise. For those with one or two mild or moderate gut symptoms, you may find this chapter is enough to rid yourself of them entirely. For others with more complex issues or stubborn symptoms, you may need a little extra support and some more investigation, which we'll walk through step by step in the coming chapters. That said, it's worth keeping an open mind – I've had many patients with debilitating symptoms regain complete control of their lives with the strategies outlined in this chapter alone. This is why I encourage everyone to start here. Even if it's not successful, it's never a waste of time; think of it instead as taking you a step closer to finding the right strategies for you and your gut. Don't worry, we're here to get you two sorted.

CHAPTER 5

Food intolerances

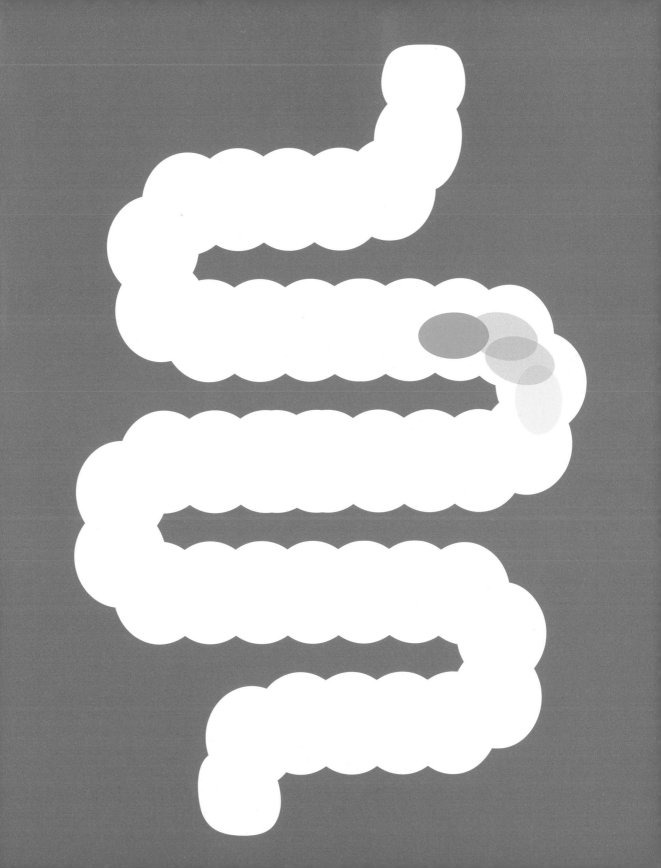

Food intolerances

Most of my patients associate their gut symptoms with eating. But once we delve a little deeper, it's only a few who turn out to have food-specific symptoms such as a food intolerance. So how do you know whether a specific food or component really doesn't agree with you or whether there is actually another cause for your gut symptoms, such as irritable bowel syndrome (IBS)? I'm not going to tell you it's straightforward, because it's not, but what makes it more difficult is all the unnecessary confusion on this topic. As a result, people tend to exclude various foods with no real coherent plan, and this can end up doing more harm than good.

One of my patients, thirty-one-year-old Stephanie, recently suffered the damaging consequences that can occur when this happens. Stephanie had been battling with gut issues since her high-school days, but after giving birth the previous year the symptoms had become so bad she was no longer able to control her bowels and, after an embarrassing incident, she was scared to leave the house. At her wits' end, Stephanie turned to online forums in a desperate attempt to resolve her debilitating symptoms. Following online advice, Stephanie began excluding different food groups such as wholegrains and dairy. Week by week, she found herself cutting out more and more suspected food culprits, until she was down to just twelve 'safe' foods. By this stage, she had become so dangerously thin that her milk supply had stopped, her once-lustrous hair had become thin and dull, her thoughts were foggy and she was on the verge of being too weak to care for her baby. At rock bottom, she came to see me in clinic. We sat together and went through her journey and, halfway through, it became abundantly clear to me that Stephanie's symptoms weren't the result of any food intolerance. Instead, she had a severe case of IBS that was being perpetuated by anxiety and malnutrition.

Yes, Stephanie's case was extreme but, sadly, this type of downward spiral with suspected food intolerances is something I see all too often in clinic.

This chapter will help cut through the confusion, equipping you with the tools and confidence to safely determine whether or not a specific food may be causing your gut symptoms.

There are two main types of food hypersensitivities: food intolerances and food allergies. Although this chapter will focus on food intolerances, it's worth knowing a little more about allergies because the two conditions are often confused with each other. Unlike food intolerances, food allergies involve the immune system, where the body mistakenly tags specific food proteins as harmful. In turn, this triggers the body's defence system. As a result, the symptoms associated with a food allergy are typically more severe than those of food intolerances and can include difficulty breathing, a racing heart rate and skin rashes as well as digestive issues. Food allergies are less common, affecting around 1 to 2 per cent of adults, and should be diagnosed only by a suitably qualified clinician. The most common food allergens are cow's milk, egg, wheat, soy, nuts, seeds and fish, although most are outgrown in early childhood. In adults, the most common form of food allergy is pollen-food syndrome. Another condition that may be considered a type of food hypersensitivity is coeliac disease. Although it involves the immune system, it is not actually an allergy but an autoimmune condition where, when exposed to gluten (a protein found in grains like wheat), the body's defence system attacks the intestine.

Food intolerances are far more common than food allergies and coeliac disease combined, affecting as many as 20 per cent of adults. Although they're not life-threatening, food intolerances can significantly impact your quality of life as well as your relationship with food, so it is worth getting on top of them.

Pollen-food syndrome (PFS)

Pollen-food syndrome (PFS), also known as oral allergy syndrome (OAS), is the single most common type of food allergy in adults. Typically, the symptoms are immediate and include mild itching, tingling or swelling of the tongue and lips. Those who get hay fever in the spring are more likely to have PFS because their body mistakes the culprit food proteins for pollen proteins and sets up an allergic response. Foods most likely to trigger symptoms include apple, kiwi, peaches, plums, carrots, Brazil nuts, walnuts, strawberries, hazelnuts and almonds. Interestingly, cooking or processing foods (e.g. canning them) may improve tolerance. This is because heating the food breaks down the protein molecules and makes them inactive so they no longer trigger an allergic reaction. Symptoms may also be relieved with antihistamines. Thankfully, PFS is not life-threatening, and in fact many people live happy, healthy lives with PFS without even realizing they have it. If you suspect you have it and it's bothering you, visit your health-care professional, who can provide further guidance on diagnosis and management.

Is it a food intolerance?

With the growing awareness of gut disorders like IBS, it's increasingly common for people to jump to the conclusion that their problem must be IBS, without considering whether their symptoms are the result of a food intolerance (the opposite of Stephanie's case). In such instances, food intolerances are left undiagnosed, which leads to ineffective management and ongoing suffering. This is why it is worth ruling out common food intolerances as a cause of your gut symptoms first. The good news is it's something you can get started with at home, using my simple 3R Method.

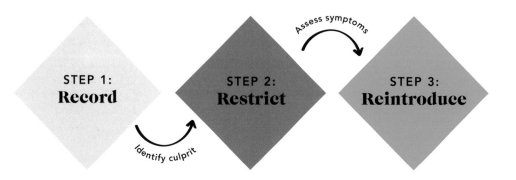

Before we make a start, I want you to remember all the good that food does for us: it gives us energy to follow our dreams and provides us with vital nutrients for our brain, hair, skin and teeth. When talking about food intolerances, it can be easy to develop negative thoughts about food. The purpose of this chapter is in fact to counter this; it's about developing your confidence and enabling you to regain the simple pleasure of eating by teaching you how to safely identify or discount a food intolerance, and so avoid unnecessary restrictions.

When it comes to symptoms, food intolerances can be expressed not only in the gut; they may also affect the skin, airways, muscles and joints and can cause headaches and fatigue. However, gut symptoms are by far the most common and will be our main focus in this chapter.

The challenges

Identifying specific food intolerances is not always straightforward. To help you become a better food-intolerance 'detective', understanding some of the main challenges can be really insightful, particularly when it comes to interpreting your results from **Step 1: Record**.

- **CHALLENGE 1:** Food is complex. Food components that can cause reactions are often naturally present in (or added to) a wide range of foods, and of course meals contain multiple ingredients. To help you overcome this challenge, I have developed tables detailing which foods and drinks contain commonly suspected culprits. If after Step 1: Record (see page 123), you're still not able to identify a food trigger using these tables but feel your symptoms are related to a food intolerance, it is possible that there is more than one culprit (although much less common). If this is the case, it's worth discussing your findings with a trained food detective – a dietitian.

- **CHALLENGE 2:** Unlike food allergies, food intolerances are often dose-dependent. This means most people with food intolerances can tolerate a portion of the food culprit. The amount (your tolerance threshold) also differs from person to person.

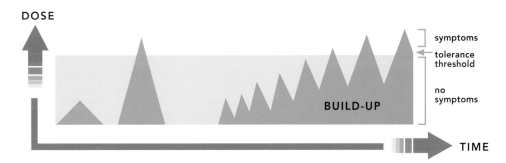

- **CHALLENGE 3:** Timing of symptoms. Symptoms experienced during or immediately after eating may have nothing to do with the meal you're eating or have just eaten. Instead, they may be related to an earlier meal. How? As we touched on in Chapter 1, when food enters the stomach it triggers movement in the large intestine, known as the gastrocolic reflex. This process helps to move previous meals through the large intestine, making them available to our hungry gut microbiota (GM). For some intolerances, this mechanism may trigger symptoms. However, for some people with IBS, it might simply be the size of the meal that triggers gut symptoms and have nothing to do with the actual food. What's more, the effect may be heightened, depending on your stress levels that day.

The common culprits

Below, we'll address the most commonly reported food intolerances that can lead to gut symptoms, including lactose (milk sugar), wheat and gluten. We'll also touch on others that you may have come across, including fructose (fruit sugar), caffeine, histamine and sulphite intolerances.

Lactose

Lactose is a unique carbohydrate found only in milk from mammals, that is, cow, goat, sheep, buffalo and human breast milk. Without wanting to bring back dreaded memories of high-school chemistry, lactose is made up of two sugars, glucose and galactose. For lactose to be absorbed from the intestine and into your bloodstream it needs to be broken down into these two single sugars. This is the job of an enzyme called lactase which is found on the lining of the small intestine. A large percentage of adults don't make enough lactase and therefore the lactose isn't absorbed efficiently in the small intestine. The prevalence of lactose intolerance varies widely between populations. For instance, lactase deficiency occurs in as few as 5 per cent of North Europeans and North Americans of European origin, yet up to 90 per cent of Asian, African and Caribbean adult populations are affected. Despite the high rates of lactase deficiency, only a subset of people actually experience gut upset and are therefore considered lactose intolerant. Why is that? For some, their GM is thought to make up for the lack of lactase enzymes by efficiently metabolizing the lactose for them.

There is some evidence suggesting that other components in standard cow's milk – specifically, certain types of protein known as A1 and A2 beta-casein – may be poorly tolerated by some people. Early-stage evidence suggests that milk with only A2 beta-casein may be better tolerated in a subset of people than milk containing a mix of the two proteins. If you live in Europe, the United States, Australia or New Zealand, the standard cow's milk typically comes from Holstein Friesian (black-and-white) cows and contains a mix of the two proteins. In contrast, cows in other areas such as Africa and India (*Bos indicus*) produce only A2 protein in their milk. We'll explore milk intolerance more in Step 3: Reintroduction.

Common symptoms associated with lactose intolerance:

- **LOOSE POOPS AND DIARRHOEA**
  (Note: This is not always the case; some may get constipation)

- **BLOATING**

- **WIND**

- **TUMMY PAIN**

TWO MAIN FORMS OF LACTOSE INTOLERANCE

1. **PRIMARY LACTASE DEFICIENCY:** This is the inherited form and typically presents between the ages of five and twenty years as lactase production decreases. This is the more common form of lactose intolerance.

2. **SECONDARY LACTASE DEFICIENCY:** As a result of a gut illness or damage to the small intestine, there is a loss of lactase production, meaning there are fewer enzymes available to digest the lactose. This, therefore, leads to malabsorption. Examples of causes include gut infections, undiagnosed coeliac disease and active Crohn's disease. The good news is that most often this type is short term. Within a few months, once the intestine has healed, the levels of lactase return to normal.

Wheat and gluten

Wheat is often the first thing to be excluded when people suspect a food intolerance. Although it's certainly not as common as suggested online, there are several wheat-related culprits that people may react to, and guess what? It's not only gluten. It's true that some people struggle to digest gluten, but there are other types of components in wheat, including wheatgerm agglutinin, amylase trypsin inhibitors and fructans, that may trigger people's symptoms. In fact, researchers have suggested that non-coeliac gluten sensitivity (NCGS) may be more accurately termed non-coeliac wheat sensitivity (NCWS), in recognition that it's not always the gluten component of wheat that people are struggling with. The jury is still out.

Why am I telling you this? I don't have a soft spot for gluten and I certainly don't want to complicate the matter, but it's worth knowing that, if you react to wheat, it may not be gluten but other components that are causing you grief. This means that not only could you be unnecessarily restricting your diet by using a gluten-free approach, but also that you won't completely shake your symptoms if the true culprit remains in your diet. This concept was demonstrated in a study where people with self-diagnosed NCGS already on a gluten-free diet further benefited when fructans (which are also found in gluten-free foods) were restricted. This is something I often see in my clinic too.

One case that particularly springs to mind is that of twenty-two-year-old James. James had self-diagnosed NCGS and, as a result, was following a strict gluten-free diet. As soon as he walked into my clinic room I could see by his hunched shoulders and negative expression that he was feeling defeated. He sat down and shared at length the struggles and hurdles he'd had to overcome to go gluten-free, including the social isolation, for example not being able to drink beer with his mates (due to standard beer containing gluten). Despite all this effort, his gut symptoms were persisting. Together, we went through his diet and I noticed he was having very large amounts of fructans, specifically from onion and garlic (fructans are a type of fermentable carbohydrate found in wheat, onions, garlic and many fruits and vegetables – we'll cover this in Chapter 6). James's symptoms suggested that he was suffering with classic IBS and so I asked him if he would be willing to cut out the onion and garlic for two weeks and report back. I could see he was a little hesitant to further restrict his diet, but after I had explained the potential mechanisms (he was studying science, after all) he was on board. Two weeks later I received an email from a very chuffed James – it had worked: his bowels, which he'd been suffering with for over three years, were no longer unruly. I did make sure that James came back to discuss reintroducing gluten-containing foods, as well as onion and garlic and other high-fructan foods, once he had better control of his IBS – oh, and the beer, now it was back on the 'menu': we did have a chat around responsible drinking too, of course!

TAKE-HOME MESSAGE: *Don't assume it's gluten and cut all sources from your diet before considering alternative causes. Step 1 in the 3R Method (see page 123) can help you objectively assess this.*

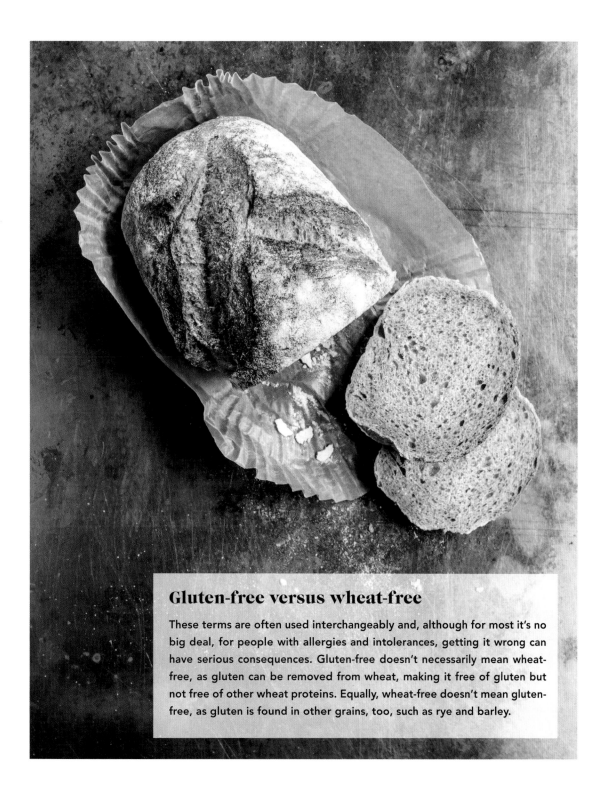

Gluten-free versus wheat-free

These terms are often used interchangeably and, although for most it's no big deal, for people with allergies and intolerances, getting it wrong can have serious consequences. Gluten-free doesn't necessarily mean wheat-free, as gluten can be removed from wheat, making it free of gluten but not free of other wheat proteins. Equally, wheat-free doesn't mean gluten-free, as gluten is found in other grains, too, such as rye and barley.

Fructose

Fructose is one of the sugars naturally found in fruit and honey. It's also increasingly being added to sweeten other food and drinks in the form of high-fructose corn syrup (HFCS), particularly in the US. Unlike the milk sugar lactose, the fruit sugar fructose is a single unit, so it doesn't need to be digested by enzymes before being absorbed into the body. On face value, you may think this means absorption is unlimited, but there is a catch: there is a quota limiting the amount of fructose that gets in at each sitting – think of it as similar to admissions into a theatre. Beyond this quota, the excess fructose has no choice but to travel onward into the large intestine, bringing with it a load of extra fluid, and is rapidly fermented by our GM. Interestingly, most of us cannot absorb large amounts of fructose in a single sitting. This explains why, when you can't stop eating those juicy cherries, even those of us with strong guts may experience some bloating and loose poops. For a subset of people, smaller amounts of fructose can trigger gut symptoms, including bloating and loose poops. Nonetheless, fructose intolerance on its own is thought to be rather rare. Instead, for those with IBS, fructose forms part of a collection of fermentable carbohydrates known as FODMAPs, which in moderate amounts may trigger symptoms in some (we'll discuss these on page 145). The good news is, if glucose is also present in the food, as in the case of most fruits, it will help your body absorb the fructose (opening a second viewing room, in the metaphor of the theatre). This is why, although all fruits contain fructose, some are better tolerated than others in people who are more sensitive, as we'll discuss when we address FODMAPs. It's also worth noting that, once you get your IBS under control, most people can enjoy higher-fructose foods without any issues.

Histamine intolerance

This can cause a range of symptoms beyond the gut. Indeed, many mimic an allergic reaction and therefore allergies should be ruled out before exploring a histamine intolerance. It can be difficult to diagnose histamine intolerance, as diet is not the only source; our body and GM can also produce histamine. Foods high in histamines include aged and fermented food and drinks (e.g. cheese, sauerkraut, alcoholic drinks, cured meats); most fish, including smoked and tinned; fruit, such as oranges and bananas; vegetables, including tomatoes, pumpkin and broad beans.

Sulphite sensitivity

Sulphite is primarily used as a preservative in a range of foods including dried fruit, processed meats and drinks, including cordials (check labels for additive numbers E220–228). They're also naturally present in fermented grape produce (i.e. wine and vinegar). People with asthma seem to have a higher risk of sensitivity. Symptoms are not gut specific and can include hives, flushing, wheezing and a stuffy nose.

Caffeine

Although most adults can consume up to 400 milligrams of caffeine a day without side effects (200mg in pregnancy), some people are more sensitive. This is related both to genetics and how it's broken down by your body. The most common side effects include nervousness, anxiety, insomnia and gut symptoms. Although we typically associate caffeine with just coffee, there are many other sources of caffeine outlined in the table below. The caffeine content isn't typically declared on food and drink labels, making it difficult to know exactly how much you are having. What makes it even more tricky is that with naturally occurring sources, such as coffee and tea, the caffeine content can vary according to the plant variety, growing conditions and brewing method. Keep this in mind when you're playing food detective.

Caffeine content of common products

BEVERAGE (serving size)	RANGE (mg)	AVERAGE (mg)
Tea		
Black (240ml)	25–110	50
Green (240ml)	30–50	45
Brewed (240ml)	40–120	55
Coffee		
Decaffeinated (240ml)	5–10	5
Instant (240ml)	25–175	95
Brewed (240ml)	100–200	135
Espresso (60ml)	60–180	80
Dark Chocolate 70% (50mg)	–	40
Cola (330ml)	10–70	40
Energy Drink (500ml)	55–175	160
Cold or Flu Medication	15–200	see packet

Source: Journal of Food Science & Food Standards Agency

Risky business

Before we get into the 3R Method, it would be remiss of me not to highlight the risks associated with a restricted diet. Long-term food restriction can not only be socially isolating, but cutting out food groups can also displace other nutrients in your diet. Take, for instance, restricting gluten. An observational study of close to 200,000 people (without coeliac disease) demonstrated that those with the highest gluten consumption (the top 20 per cent) had a 20 per cent lower risk of developing type 2 diabetes, compared to those with the lowest gluten intake (the bottom 20 per cent). When the researchers delved further into it, they were able to explain this finding, at least in part, by the fact that those who cut gluten were also tending to eat less grain fibre; grain fibre is known to protect against type 2 diabetes. What about our GM? It's affected too. For instance, a gluten-free diet has been shown to decrease certain bacteria known to produce those beneficial short-chain fatty acids (SCFA).

Still not convinced about these knock-on effects? Researchers have shown that not only were gluten-free foods 159 per cent more expensive, they also, on average, contained more added sugar and salt, and less fibre and protein, compared to their gluten-containing alternatives. Now, of course, opting for more whole foods and less processed options (e.g. choosing gluten-free oats instead of ultra-processed gluten-free cereals) can help to avoid this when going gluten-free. It does, however, highlight the need to be more aware of the ways in which other aspects of your diet can be affected if you cut foods out. Long-term food restriction may also lead to greater sensitivity to certain foods too. Considering all these factors, it becomes rather apparent that restricting your diet when you don't need to may do more harm than good.

 Caution: If you have a history of disordered eating, please seek support from a dietitian before considering the 3R Method.

Diagnosing intolerances

The gold standard for diagnosing food intolerances is an exclusion diet, followed by a placebo-controlled reintroduction. These describe Step 2 and Step 3 in the 3R Method, respectively. This is based on a simple rationale: restriction of the food component under suspicion should resolve your symptoms, and reintroduction should reproduce symptoms.

When it comes to Step 3, it's recommended that this is done blinded, which means that you are unaware of whether you are eating the challenge food or a placebo (a food without the suspected culprit). This comes back to the gut–brain axis. Remember: the communication between the two is bidirectional, meaning the gut can influence the brain, and vice versa. Studies have shown that if we perceive that we have a food intolerance, our brain can send messages to our gut inducing gut symptoms when we eat the suspected culprit. This phenomenon is known as the nocebo effect – the ability of negative expectations to manifest physical symptoms. Need the science to convince you? Don't worry: I did, too. A systematic review (that's where scientists pool together the results from all the trials on one topic) found that 40 per cent of people with a self-reported intolerance to gluten had similar or increased symptoms during the placebo (i.e. gluten-free) intervention, because they believed it contained gluten. It's similar to when we are mentally stressed or nervous: it can physically manifest into gut symptoms, despite our diet not changing. These findings reinforce why we shouldn't underestimate the power of our thoughts.

Invalid food tolerances

Despite the convincing marketing claims, there is no valid test for food intolerances (with lactose being the exception). Some of the common invalid tests to watch out for include IgG tests, hair analysis and muscle analysis (kinesiology). Many of these tests attach themselves to scientific concepts that sound rather convincing. Take, for instance, the IgG tests. This test involves exposing a sample of your blood to different foods and measuring the resulting antibody (IgG). The test claims this is a marker of 'intolerance'. Sounds pretty legit, right? The thing is, unlike IgE which are valid for diagnosing certain allergies, most of us will actually develop IgG antibodies to food during our lifetime, despite not getting symptoms. This, explains expert immunologist Dr Macciochi, is because IgG is an indicator of repeated exposure, not a food intolerance.

The 3R Method

There is no denying that food intolerances can be confusing to navigate, which is why the medical guidelines recommend seeing a dietitian. But having worked in both public and private sectors of health care, I know access to a dietitian is not always straightforward, with long waiting lists (and cost in the private sector) a deterrent for many. For those with only mild symptoms, it may also seem a little too much as a first step. So what do we instinctively do? Turn to Google, of course. The outcome? Conflicting advice, long-term over-restriction and persisting symptoms as you're sucked into a downhill spiral, like Stephanie. The answer? I'm going to be straight and tell you there's no quick fix. But there is a more effective and safer way of going about it – the 3R Method. This is something I developed with you guys in mind. The purpose is to provide you with the evidence-based tools needed to start the detective work safely at home. It's also the framework I regularly use in my clinic, as was the case with thirty-one-year-old Karen.

Karen had been suffering with bloating, loose poops and bowel urgency since her early twenties. She explained that she'd recently been told that she had IBS and, after reading about the benefits of a low-FODMAP diet, wanted to give it a try. I did my normal work-up and found that Karen didn't fulfil the criteria for IBS (we'll discuss this in Chapter 6). Furthermore, from her brief diet history (her two-year-old son was getting a little impatient with us), I found that Karen's diet was really rather low in FODMAPs. I explained these findings to her, along with the complexity of the low-FODMAP diet, and suggested instead that, as a first step, we investigated whether a food tolerance could be the cause. Karen was, not surprisingly, a little relieved at not having to follow a strict diet. She also explained that she'd considered dairy and gluten intolerance over the years but cutting them out never seemed to solve things. I asked Karen to complete Step 1: Record, and return in a few weeks.

In order for you to play food detective, you need to collect some objective information. This involves recording a detailed diary for seven days, or two weeks if symptoms are less frequent, as outlined overleaf. If you're confident that you've already identified a food culprit, then you can move straight to Step 2.

During Step 1, try to keep your diet and lifestyle as normal as you can (whatever that looks like for you). This is because the purpose is to identify whether anything you normally eat or do is causing the problem. If you can, the most accurate pictures come from when you record things in real time so that you remember to include all the details, for example, that bite of your friend's burger or the leftover crisps from your staff meeting. To help with this, it's a good idea to carry your diary with you (or use a smartphone tracker app).

Main sources of commonly reported food intolerances:

- **LACTOSE:** Milk from animals, soft cheeses, yoghurt and milk-based desserts, e.g. custard and ice cream.

- **WHEAT:** All types (e.g. durum, farro, spelt, einkorn, kamut and triticiale) and forms (e.g. semolina, couscous) of wheat.

- **GLUTEN:** All foods containing rye, wheat or barley, e.g. breakfast cereals, bread, pizza, pasta, cake; and beer, barley squash and malted drinks.

My Gut Diary

This diary is designed to capture your gut symptoms, along with the key factors that can influence them, like diet, mood, sleep, pooping habits and other activities. The more accurate your diary is, the more helpful it will be in getting on top of your gut symptoms. You might like to use the diary template from www.TheGutHealthDoctor.com or just convert a small notepad into your diary. Here are some tips for completing it:

1. **WRITE DOWN EVERYTHING YOU EAT AND DRINK,** and the time (remember to record those easily forgotten things like chewing gum, supplements, medication, total fluid intake, and so on).

2. **TRY TO BE SPECIFIC,** including condiments like sauces and spreads, how it was cooked (e.g. fried or raw), and estimated portions (no need to get the scales out). Write clearly, in case you need to share it with your dietitian.

3. **RECORD DETAILS OF THE SYMPTOMS,** including the time they started, the duration and the severity. Use the scale 1 (mild) to 5 (severe) to capture the severity.

4. **RECORD OTHER EVENTS AND ACTIVITIES,** including exercise, stressors such as work meetings or family arguments, general mood, bedtime, waking time, pooping habits and so on.

Karen returned three weeks later, having dutifully completed her gut diary – it was time to play food detective. Karen's symptoms were worse during the week, on days she had a wheat-based breakfast cereal (with soy milk). From her diary, I could also see that each time she'd eaten a 50 gram chocolate bar or custard she'd have bowel urgency within an hour. After piecing together the information, I suspected that it was lactose. But what about her breakfast – she was using lactose-free milk after all? Unknown to Karen, her breakfast cereal wasn't lactose-free as it contained skimmed-milk powder (a marketing trick to boost the protein and sweetness). I also noticed that she was taking a high-dose vitamin C supplement (she'd read it was a flu preventative).

With these clues noted, Karen moved on to Step 2, implementing three changes: 1. cutting out high-lactose foods (see page 129); 2. stopping her vitamin C supplement (which at a high dose can cause gut upset); and 3. increasing her fruit intake (high in vitamin C) to two pieces spread across the day (Karen had cut out fruit, as she'd heard it was high in sugar and caused candida overgrowth – I happily busted that myth for her).

Now it's your turn to play detective using your diary.
Follow the flow diagram below to determine the next step for you.

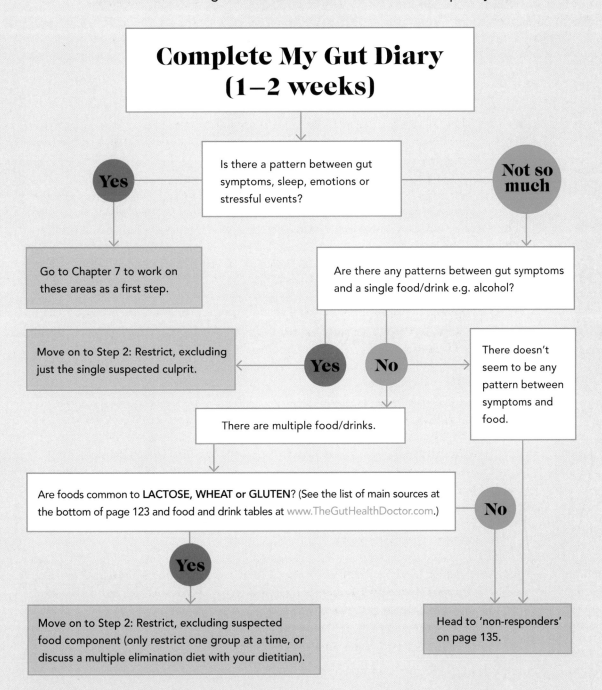

Complete My Gut Diary (1–2 weeks)

Is there a pattern between gut symptoms, sleep, emotions or stressful events?

Yes → Go to Chapter 7 to work on these areas as a first step.

Not so much → Are there any patterns between gut symptoms and a single food/drink e.g. alcohol?

Yes → Move on to Step 2: Restrict, excluding just the single suspected culprit.

No → There are multiple food/drinks.

There doesn't seem to be any pattern between symptoms and food.

Are foods common to **LACTOSE, WHEAT or GLUTEN**? (See the list of main sources at the bottom of page 123 and food and drink tables at www.TheGutHealthDoctor.com.)

Yes → Move on to Step 2: Restrict, excluding suspected food component (only restrict one group at a time, or discuss a multiple elimination diet with your dietitian).

No → Head to 'non-responders' on page 135.

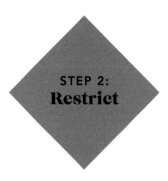

STEP 2:
Restrict

So, your suspected food culprit (or culprits) has been identified – what next? As discussed earlier, the more you restrict it, the greater the nutritional risk. Therefore, if you have identified multiple food culprits (e.g. lactose and wheat), it's recommended that you see a dietitian who can help guide you through restricting several food components at once. Also, remember: if you suspect an issue with gluten or wheat, it is best to see your doctor to be tested for coeliac disease *before* excluding it from your diet. Why? You need to include a considerable amount of gluten in the diet for at least six weeks in order for your coeliac test to be valid.

PREPARATION IS KEY. RESTRICTING COMMON FOODS CAN TAKE SOME PLANNING.

- **TIME:** Choose a convenient period. Avoiding busy times at work and peak social seasons will make it easier to stick to the restrictions. If you do eat the food by mistake or for social reasons, it's completely okay. Just know that you may have residual symptoms for up to three days or so.

- **KNOWLEDGE:** Take a week or so to become familiar with dietary sources and the suggested alternative foods to ensure your diet is still nutritionally adequate. This is not a 'detox' or weight-loss diet; you should still be meeting all your nutritional requirements and not excluding whole food groups.

- **CLEAN OUT AND RESTOCK:** Donate to a food bank or use up any foods you plan to restrict, and buy the alternative replacements.

- **HABIT-FORMING:** Get into the habit of checking labels before you start and consider planning meals for your first week to help ease yourself into it.

- **SUPPORT:** Keep your family and friends in the loop so they can help support you.

FOR EACH OF THE COMMON INTOLERANCES, YOU WILL FIND A TABLE AT www.TheGutHealthDoctor.com **OUTLINING:**

1. **FOODS AND DRINKS TO RESTRICT AND THEIR ALTERNATIVES:** This should be used to help guide your dietary choices to ensure you are not cutting out whole food groups. Keep in mind that these tables are not complete lists and suitability may differ between brands. It's best to always check the product label.

2. **INGREDIENT NAMES ON FOOD LABELS TO WATCH OUT FOR:** Suspected food components are often added as ingredients to foods and drinks, some of which you may not expect (such as the skimmed-milk powder in Karen's breakfast cereal). If the product contains any of the ingredients listed in the table, it is best avoided during Step 2 for simplicity, although remember, you will be able to tolerate small amounts, even if intolerant, because it's not an allergy. How much exactly? That will be dictated by your tolerance threshold, which we'll assess in Step 3: Reintroduce.

3. **NUTRIENTS TO WATCH:** Restricting foods can have a knock-on effect in terms of your micronutrient intake. To ensure you're still meeting all your nutritional needs, make sure to include alternative sources of the nutrients listed.

Before you remove the suspected culprit from your diet, use the **Gut Feelings Assessment** from Chapter 1 (page 21) to assess your symptoms. It is then time to begin the restriction. If your symptoms resolve after two weeks, you can move straight on to Step 3 – there is no need to wait. If, by week four, your symptoms have improved slightly, you may wish to continue up to of six weeks before moving on to Step 3. If your symptoms don't improve at all after four weeks, or only slightly after six weeks, it is best to put the eliminated food back into your diet and return to your usual diet. From there, head to page 135 – Step 3 is not relevant to your situation.

How did Karen get on? Her symptoms vanished after just one week. She couldn't believe it was that 'simple'. She was kicking herself for not having taken a more systematic approach when dealing with her initial suspicion of a food intolerance. The next step was reintroducing and, although a little apprehensive, Karen understood it was best to confirm it really was the lactose and high-dose vitamin C causing the problem. Karen challenged them one by one.

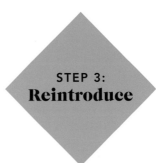

STEP 3:
Reintroduce

This step is essential to confirm whether the suspect food component really is the cause of your gut symptoms and not just an innocent bystander. It will also help you determine your tolerance threshold. If you have any concerns that it is an allergy, see your GP or allergy specialist first and do not reintroduce. For those tempted to skip this section and just restrict the food long term, here are some points worth considering.

- **UNNECESSARILY OVER-RESTRICTING YOUR DIET INCREASES YOUR RISK OF MALNUTRITION,** which occurs when your body doesn't get enough nutrients to maintain itself and your muscles start to waste. This can leave you feeling tired and more likely to catch the flu, among many other things.

- **COMPLETE RESTRICTION OVER A LONG PERIOD OF TIME MAY INCREASE YOUR SENSITIVITY,** that is, lower your tolerance threshold. As a consequence, symptoms may increase in severity when you accidentally eat those foods. I often see this with lactose intolerance.

- **A RESTRICTED DIET LONG TERM IS LINKED WITH A REDUCED FOOD-RELATED QUALITY OF LIFE,** that is, it reduces the fun of eating and socializing – and nobody wants that.

- **MANY OF THESE FOODS ARE YOUR GM'S FAVOURITES,** which means that you could not only be denying your taste buds but your GM too.

> **Caution:** If you have been avoiding a food group for several years and have history of atopic symptoms (i.e. eczema, asthma or hay fever), it is recommended that reintroduction is conducted by an allergy-specialist dietitian or an allergist.

As we touched on earlier, the reintroduction process is most accurate when you are blinded to the food, that is, you don't know whether you're having the 'active/challenge' food or the placebo test food. How to go about doing this, including test foods and amounts, is described in the flow diagrams on the next few pages. If you have identified a single food or drink culprit, follow the diagram on pages 132–33, using this as your 'test food'. On day one start with one third of your normal portion, and increase by one third each day as appropriate. For blinding, you'll need to get your family or a friend on board. Ask them to disguise the food so you can't tell the difference between the active and the placebo. Blending, toasting or crumbling can be helpful ways to blind you – although be sure they don't add in any other suspected culprits in doing so! Before you are unblinded, complete both active and placebo challenges, even if you get symptoms with the first challenge. If you do get symptoms, wait until you are symptom free again (usually up to three days) before moving on to the other test food. I get that it's not always possible to do food challenges blinded, so don't let that stop you from completing Step 3.

Lactose content of milk and dairy products

TYPE	% BY WEIGHT
Cow's Milk	4.5
Condensed Milk	12.5
Milk Powder	53.0
Goat's Milk	4.5
Sheep's Milk	5.0
Cream	2.0
Crème Fraîche	2.5
Imitation Cream	2.5–7.0
Firm Cheese e.g. Cheddar	Less than 1.0
Processed Cheese e.g. cheese spread	4.5–7.5
Cottage Cheese	3.0
Yoghurt	4.5
Ice Cream	5.0
Rice Pudding	4.0
Custard	5.0
Chocolate (milk, white)	9.0–10.0
Chocolate (dark, 70%)	Less than 1.0
Butter	Less than 1.0

Source: McCance and Widdowson

Testing response to lactose

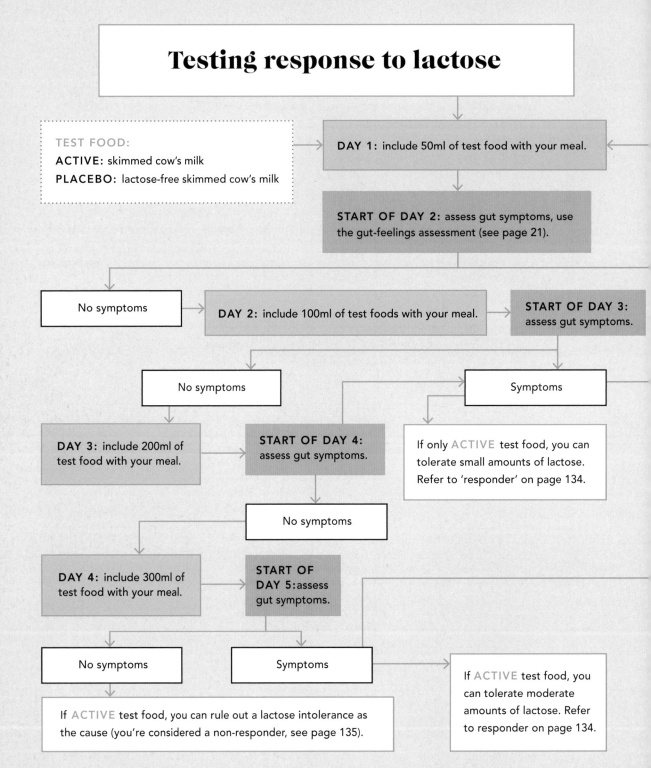

TEST FOOD:
ACTIVE: skimmed cow's milk
PLACEBO: lactose-free skimmed cow's milk

DAY 1: include 50ml of test food with your meal.

START OF DAY 2: assess gut symptoms, use the gut-feelings assessment (see page 21).

No symptoms

DAY 2: include 100ml of test foods with your meal.

START OF DAY 3: assess gut symptoms.

No symptoms

Symptoms

DAY 3: include 200ml of test food with your meal.

START OF DAY 4: assess gut symptoms.

If only ACTIVE test food, you can tolerate small amounts of lactose. Refer to 'responder' on page 134.

No symptoms

DAY 4: include 300ml of test food with your meal.

START OF DAY 5: assess gut symptoms.

No symptoms

Symptoms

If ACTIVE test food, you can rule out a lactose intolerance as the cause (you're considered a non-responder, see page 135).

If ACTIVE test food, you can tolerate moderate amounts of lactose. Refer to responder on page 134.

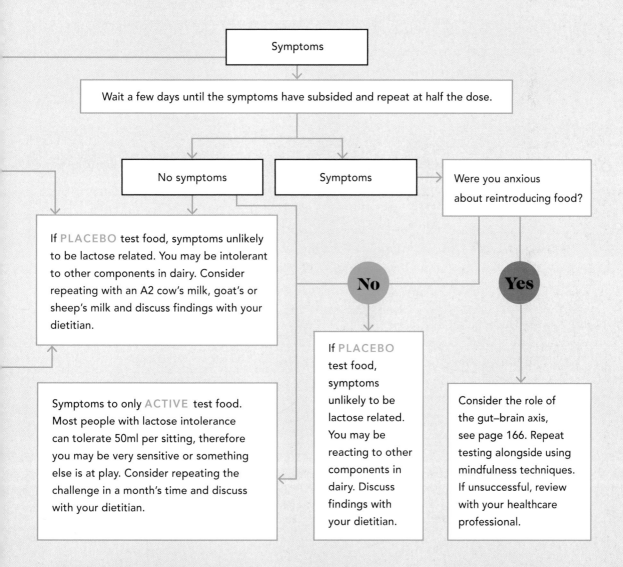

Continue a low lactose diet throughout the test period.

Symptoms

Wait a few days until the symptoms have subsided and repeat at half the dose.

No symptoms

Symptoms

Were you anxious about reintroducing food?

If PLACEBO test food, symptoms unlikely to be lactose related. You may be intolerant to other components in dairy. Consider repeating with an A2 cow's milk, goat's or sheep's milk and discuss findings with your dietitian.

No

Yes

Symptoms to only ACTIVE test food. Most people with lactose intolerance can tolerate 50ml per sitting, therefore you may be very sensitive or something else is at play. Consider repeating the challenge in a month's time and discuss with your dietitian.

If PLACEBO test food, symptoms unlikely to be lactose related. You may be reacting to other components in dairy. Discuss findings with your dietitian.

Consider the role of the gut–brain axis, see page 166. Repeat testing alongside using mindfulness techniques. If unsuccessful, review with your healthcare professional.

Testing response to gluten/wheat

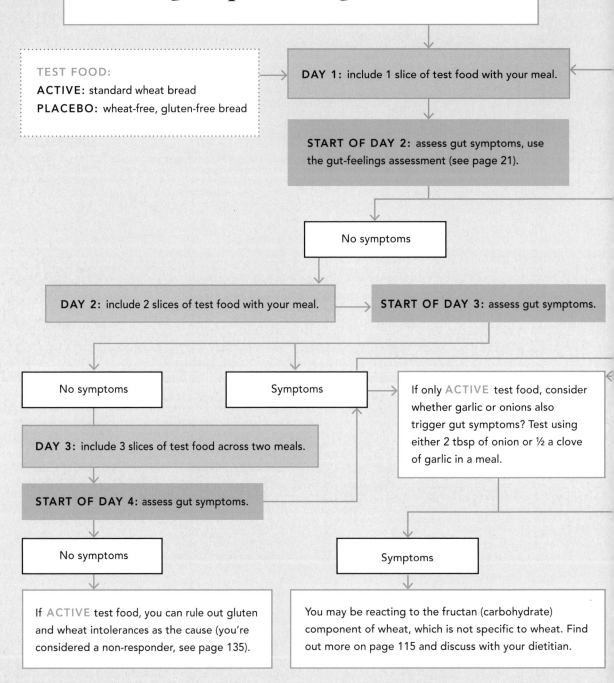

TEST FOOD:
ACTIVE: standard wheat bread
PLACEBO: wheat-free, gluten-free bread

DAY 1: include 1 slice of test food with your meal.

START OF DAY 2: assess gut symptoms, use the gut-feelings assessment (see page 21).

No symptoms

DAY 2: include 2 slices of test food with your meal.

START OF DAY 3: assess gut symptoms.

No symptoms

Symptoms

If ACTIVE test food, consider whether garlic or onions also trigger gut symptoms? Test using either 2 tbsp of onion or ½ a clove of garlic in a meal.

DAY 3: include 3 slices of test food across two meals.

START OF DAY 4: assess gut symptoms.

No symptoms

Symptoms

If ACTIVE test food, you can rule out gluten and wheat intolerances as the cause (you're considered a non-responder, see page 135).

You may be reacting to the fructan (carbohydrate) component of wheat, which is not specific to wheat. Find out more on page 115 and discuss with your dietitian.

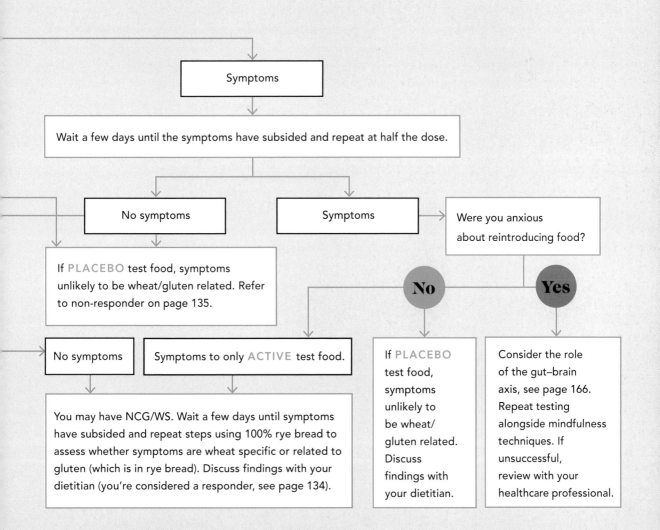

Continue a gluten/wheat-free diet throughout the test period.

Symptoms

Wait a few days until the symptoms have subsided and repeat at half the dose.

No symptoms

Symptoms

Were you anxious about reintroducing food?

If PLACEBO test food, symptoms unlikely to be wheat/gluten related. Refer to non-responder on page 135.

No

Yes

No symptoms

Symptoms to only ACTIVE test food.

You may have NCG/WS. Wait a few days until symptoms have subsided and repeat steps using 100% rye bread to assess whether symptoms are wheat specific or related to gluten (which is in rye bread). Discuss findings with your dietitian (you're considered a responder, see page 134).

If PLACEBO test food, symptoms unlikely to be wheat/gluten related. Discuss findings with your dietitian.

Consider the role of the gut–brain axis, see page 166. Repeat testing alongside mindfulness techniques. If unsuccessful, review with your healthcare professional.

What next?

FOR THE RESPONDERS: If it turns out that you're intolerant to one of the common culprits, bear in mind that it may not be for ever. This is why reassessing your tolerances over time is a good idea. If you find that you can tolerate small amounts of the food, then it is advisable to continue to include the foods up to your tolerance threshold (particularly for lactose). If you do feel it's necessary to exclude them completely, remember to nourish your body with the other sources of the key nutrients to ensure your diet remains balanced. If ever in doubt, be sure to see a dietitian or registered nutritionist.

Can you increase your tolerance threshold? There is some evidence to suggest you can, particularly for lactose, as outlined below. If you have issues with wheat, but also find that you have IBS (see Chapter 6), once your IBS is under control you may find you can reintroduce larger portions of wheat.

Improving tolerance to lactose

- *Most can continue to eat small amounts across the day without symptoms (up to 12g lactose/day).*

- *Consume as part of a meal rather than on its own.*

- *Consuming small amounts regularly may help increase your tolerance (possibly through adaptation of your GM – it may even act as a prebiotic).*

- *Fermented milk products, including live yoghurt and kefir, typically contain less lactose compared to equivalent non-fermented forms, thanks to the microbes which eat some of it. Keep in mind that the amount varies, depending on the types of microbes and the time left to ferment.*

FOR NON-RESPONDERS: For those who didn't identify any food triggers, I appreciate that you may feel somewhat disheartened that you haven't got to the bottom of your issue at this stage, but please don't be. There are a number of positive outcomes that have resulted from going through this systematic process. First, if you were restricting foods, you should now be able to confidently reintroduce them, knowing that they aren't the cause. Second, for some, Step 1 may have helped you identify other non-diet-related triggers such as stress, which can be managed by adopting the strategies we'll discuss in Chapter 7. Third, ruling out these common food intolerances will have you better placed to move on to Chapter 6 and assess whether, like in Stephanie's case, IBS could in fact be behind your symptoms. Fourth, if you still suspect a food intolerance, having gone through the three steps will make the next step (seeing your health-care professional) much more efficient in helping you to identify what lies at the root of your gut issues. How? You've already completed the first-line strategies that your GP or dietitian would normally spend the first appointment addressing, allowing them to move on to investigating more complex causes. Along with taking your completed My Gut Diary to your appointment, it's always a good idea to prepare yourself for the questions you may be asked in your appointment so you can get the most out of your time with them (see below).

- Do your symptoms follow a pattern, for example, are they always in the evening?

- Have you had any previous tests or examinations?

- Are your symptoms affected by stress?

- How quickly after eating do you see a reaction?

- Do you have a family history of gut issues, allergies or any other conditions?

- What is your most troublesome symptom?

- When did your symptoms first start?

- How often do you experience symptoms in a week or a month?

- Are you on any medication or supplements? (Best to bring a list with you, if you are.)

- Do you suffer from any allergies (e.g. eczema, asthma, hay fever, animal hair, house dust mite, other diagnosed food allergies)?

CHAPTER 6

Irritable bowel syndrome

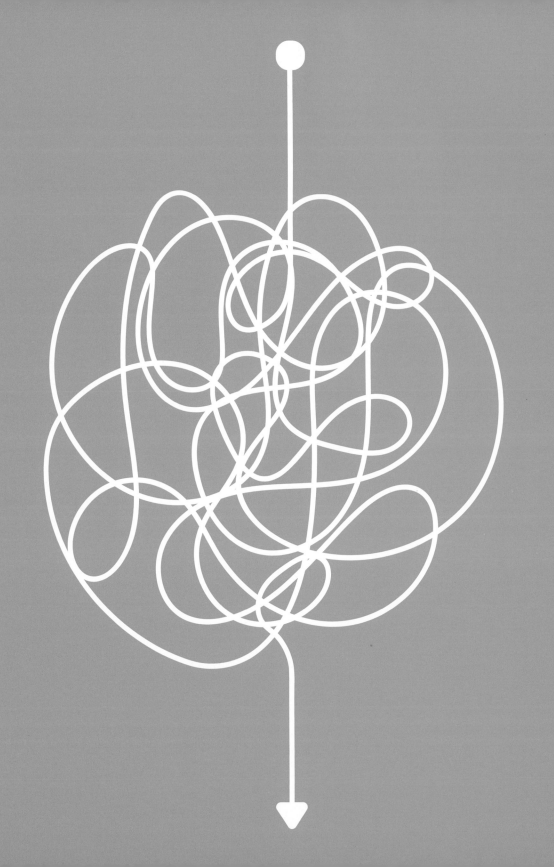

IBS

Do you suffer from several gut symptoms, including tummy pain? Having a collection of symptoms is extremely common, particularly in people with irritable bowel syndrome (IBS), a gut disorder that affects as many as one in ten adults worldwide.

For many, IBS can be extremely debilitating. It can affect your work life with more time taken off sick, your social life with more cancelled events, and your self-confidence, too, as it can cause bloating that rivals the size of a pregnant belly. What further adds to many people's frustration is the unpredictability and inability to control symptoms. Indeed, one study of nearly 2,000 IBS sufferers found that they would be willing to give up 25 per cent of their remaining lifespan to be symptom free – reinforcing just how crippling the condition can be.

> I witnessed this level of despair in forty-one-year-old Jack. Over a two-year period, Jack had seen over fifteen different specialists, travelling across the country in a desperate attempt to cure his debilitating gut symptoms. He quit his job, re-mortgaged his house and admitted that his pervasive suicidal thoughts may have ended with him taking his own life if it hadn't been for his supportive partner, who happened to be a psychologist.

While the severity of the symptoms varies from person to person, suffering with uncontrolled IBS should be a thing of the past. There are now international guidelines informing the management of IBS, along with breakthrough research, including work from my research team, highlighting the powerful role that diet can play.

For those with IBS, this chapter is about equipping you with the necessary information and tools to get you on the road to recovery, just like Jack, who was able to take control of his IBS. We will cover the evidence behind the syndrome, including what to expect, how to self-manage and when you may need to call in the gut experts.

First up, is it IBS?

This seemingly simple question is actually quite tricky, because there is currently no specific test to diagnose IBS. Instead, it's a diagnosis you and your GP come to after ruling out other diseases, such as coeliac disease and inflammatory bowel disease (IBD), where symptoms often overlap with IBS (see the red flags on page 81). Thankfully, there are simple tests your GP can perform to rule these out, which is why I always recommend paying them a visit before attributing your symptoms to IBS.

The cause:

IBS is considered a disorder of the gut–brain axis. This essentially means that the communication between the gut and the brain is out of whack, which is expressed through an overly sensitive intestine, which, as we touched on earlier, is more formally referred to as visceral hypersensitivity. As a result, there is an exaggerated response to various things, including fluctuating hormones, food and drinks and medication. This explains why most people find their symptoms get worse with poor sleep, stress and after eating and drinking.

There is no single cause for IBS; instead, several factors can increase your risk of getting it. One of the most well known is suffering from a gut infection like traveller's diarrhoea or food poisoning. In fact, your risk of getting IBS is over four times greater if you've had a gut infection in the previous year. It has also been suggested that, in addition to having a gut infection, your risk is further increased by your gender (it's higher in females), the severity of infection and a history of anxiety or depression. Interestingly, a history of trauma and chronic stress are additional risk factors for IBS. There may also be a genetic component to IBS, suggesting that some people are more susceptible than others, based on suspect genes linked to gut movement, gut 'leakiness' and how sensitive your intestine is. It might be worth chatting to your parents about whether they've ever suffered with IBS. That said, having specific genes doesn't mean you are destined for IBS; instead, it's determined by a combination of genes and your environment. For instance, stress (your environment) can affect whether IBS-related genes are 'switched on'.

Assessment: DO YOU HAVE IBS?
Head to www.TheGutHealthDoctor.com to complete the IBS assessment to determine whether you might have IBS or another functional gut disorder.

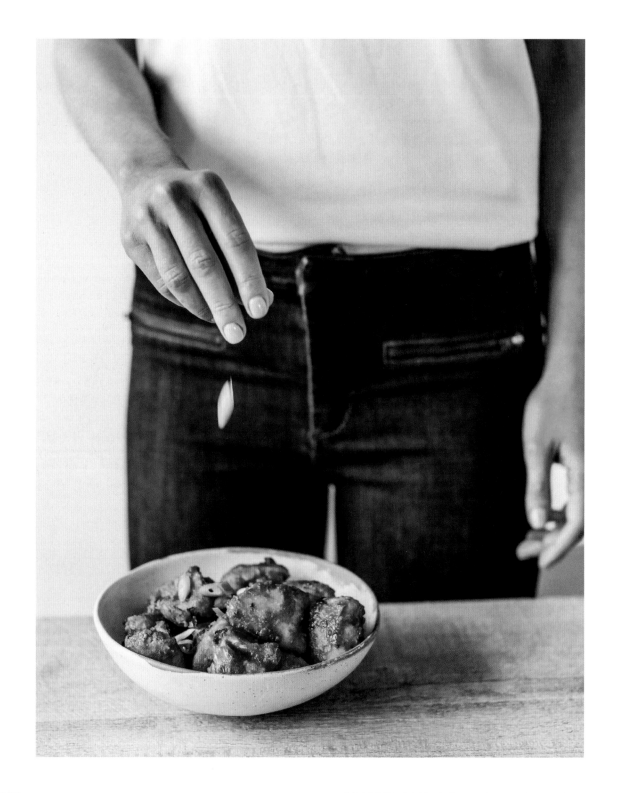

Changing up your diet

Diet has revolutionized the management of IBS, with research demonstrating that the majority of people are able to effectively manage their symptoms by making changes to what they eat and drink. This makes sense, given that around 90 per cent of people with IBS say that food triggers their symptoms. There are two main ways to tackle IBS symptoms through changes to your diet. The first-line approach has been shown to achieve impressive benefits in around 50 per cent of IBS suffers. Better still, it's something you can start on your own. The second-line approach is a little more in-depth and involves restriction of a group of carbohydrates known as FODMAPs, many of which are prebiotics, followed by staged reintroductions.

Diet can be very effective in getting your symptoms under control, but it doesn't necessarily target the underlying cause of your IBS. As a result, if diet is the only change you make, when trigger foods are reintroduced, often the symptoms also return. I see diet not as the solution but as part of the solution. Diet typically begins to take effect anywhere from a few days to a few weeks, which gives your gut time to 'rest' (as well as giving you some symptom-free sanity). It also allows time for the slower-acting complementary non-diet approaches to take effect, which I recommend you begin alongside changes in your diet. These non-diet approaches have been shown to target the disordered gut–brain communication, i.e. the underlying cause. They include sleep hygiene, mindfulness, gut-directed yoga and breathing strategies, among others. We'll go through these in detail, along with exercises for you to try, in Chapter 7.

Not everyone's IBS works in the same way, and research from my team suggests that some of these differences may explain why different people respond to different therapies. This reinforces the message that managing IBS is not a one-size-fits-all approach.

 Caution: IBS dietary advice may trigger negative thinking patterns if you have a history of an eating disorder. Best to see a dietitian for support.

First-line diet approach

It is both the *way* you eat and *what* you eat that can impact gut symptoms. This is because eating can affect gut movements, gut permeability (aka leakiness), stress hormones (yep, your diet can impact these too!) and your GM. Despite this, most of us tend to focus all our attention on what we're eating and disregard the way we eat entirely.

Take one of my patients, Dan, a thirty-two-year-old lawyer whose story is a great example of this. After Dan caught a stomach bug on holiday, his bowels were never the same. He suffered with altered bowel habits (some days diarrhoea, others constipation), excessive bloating, tummy pain and reflux for close to a year. Dan was convinced he was intolerant to a particular food but couldn't seem to pinpoint the culprit. He'd tried cutting gluten, dairy, raw foods, cooked foods, acidic foods and just about every other commonly victimized food you may read about online, but none of his attempts seemed to provide any benefit. In fact, he noticed that many of the restrictions made his symptoms worse. Dan was very diligent and came to our consultation with a typed list of all the foods he'd eaten in the previous week, along with a timeline of the symptoms he had experienced. I asked Dan to describe more about his actual eating patterns. He explained that he wasn't much of a morning person so had his first meal around noon, often on the run between meetings, and then wouldn't eat again until he got home, after 8 p.m. I probed a little further about how he ate his meals, and with that I could see he was a little confused. Why was I focusing on how he was eating rather than the food list he had so diligently prepared? Noting Dan's confusion, I walked him through how digestion worked, explaining that the sheer act of filling the stomach leads to a release of communication molecules that stimulate the bowel and affect movement, among many other things. I shared that, in some people, this can lead to discomfort soon after eating. Although a little hesitant, Dan agreed over the next four weeks to shift his focus from what he was eating to how he was eating. We agreed on two strategies: 1. to continue eating the same amount and type of food but to spread it across five eating occasions in a day; and 2. to eat only when sitting down and with technology switched off (phone, computer and television). Four weeks later, the frequency of Dan's symptoms had halved and, after adding in stress-management techniques (including mindfulness, which we look at on page 178), within two months he was back in control of his gut and his life.

So what exactly does this first-line diet approach involve? It looks at both specific components of food known to stimulate the gut and your eating pattern, as detailed across. The first step will make good use of your My Gut Diary from Chapter 5.

Dietary component	Main sources and considerations
ALCOHOL	All alcoholic drinks. Response is typically dose dependent, meaning small amounts may be okay. Ciders, sweet wines and rum may be worse because of the FODMAP content (see page 145). **RECOMMENDATION:** No more than one standard drink a day (equivalent of around 330ml low-strength beer, 100ml wine or 25ml spirit). Or, if you're up for it, go without for the four-week trial.
CAFFEINE	See page 119. **RECOMMENDATION:** Limit to one caffeine-containing drink/ food a day, e.g. 1 single shot coffee, 1 tea (limiting to 50–100mg caffeine per day). Or, if you're up for it, go without for the four-week trial.
SPICY FOOD	Any dish containing chilli. **RECOMMENDATION:** Limit chilli-containing meals.
FAT	Fried foods and fatty meats, e.g. chips, non-traditional pizzas, deep-fried chicken; pastries, cakes, chocolate, shortbread, pies, crisps; full-fat cheese, cream, coconut milk. **RECOMMENDATION:** Limit large portions of high-fat foods, particularly those with limited nutritional value, i.e. high-fat fast food.
WATER	All liquids. **RECOMMENDATION:** 1.5–2 litres of fluid per day (aim for mostly water).
DIETARY FIBRE	Fruit, vegetables, wholegrains, legumes, nuts, seeds, products fortified with fibre such as inulin and oligofructose/fructo-oligosaccharide. **RECOMMENDATION:** Spread fibre intake evenly across the day. Aim for 2 pieces of fruit, 5 portions of vegetables, 3 portions of wholegrains and 1 or 2 portions of nuts/ seeds/ legumes each day. If intake is above, reduce for the four-week trial; if below, gradually increase, as discussed on page 50.
FRUIT	Fresh, dried, juices, smoothies. **RECOMMENDATION:** No more than 1 piece of fruit per sitting (equivalent of 80g fresh or 30g dried) with up to three sittings across the day. Limit juices and smoothies, eat whole fruits.
SWEETENERS ENDING IN -OL (+ ISOMALT)	Sugar-free/ low-calorie foods, chewing gum and other food and drinks with added mannitol, maltitol, sorbitol, xylitol or isomalt. **RECOMMENDATION:** Avoid all sweeteners ending in -ol.

Follow the flow diagram below to determine the next step for you.

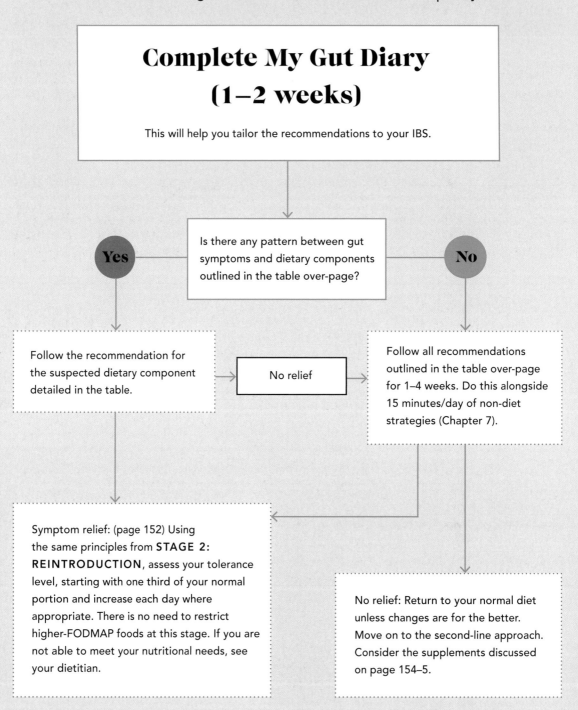

Complete My Gut Diary (1–2 weeks)

This will help you tailor the recommendations to your IBS.

Is there any pattern between gut symptoms and dietary components outlined in the table over-page?

Yes

No

Follow the recommendation for the suspected dietary component detailed in the table.

No relief

Follow all recommendations outlined in the table over-page for 1–4 weeks. Do this alongside 15 minutes/day of non-diet strategies (Chapter 7).

Symptom relief: (page 152) Using the same principles from **STAGE 2: REINTRODUCTION**, assess your tolerance level, starting with one third of your normal portion and increase each day where appropriate. There is no need to restrict higher-FODMAP foods at this stage. If you are not able to meet your nutritional needs, see your dietitian.

No relief: Return to your normal diet unless changes are for the better. Move on to the second-line approach. Consider the supplements discussed on page 154–5.

Second-line diet approach

If it turns out your IBS is a little more stubborn, this is when a low-FODMAP diet is worth considering. The low-FODMAP diet was first developed by colleagues from Monash University in Australia and is backed by a body of good-quality trials, with success seen in around 70 per cent of people.

What are FODMAPs?

FODMAPs are a group of carbohydrates found in a wide range of foods which are poorly absorbed in the small intestine. Without getting too sciencey on you, the term 'FODMAP' stands for Fermentable Oligosaccharides, Disaccharides, Monosaccharides and Polyols, which are the scientific names given to groups of carbohydrates based on their chemical structure. The table below helps break things down. Within each of these carbohydrate groups there are specific types that are restricted during the initial stage of the low-FODMAP diet.

Carbohydrate groups	Carbohydrates restricted short-term	Key dietary sources
OLIGOSACCHARIDES	Fructans [Fructo-oligosaccharides (FOS) & inulin] Galacto-oligosaccharides (GOS)	Wheat, rye, specific fruit and vegetables, e.g. onion and garlic, and added prebiotics Legumes such as kidney beans
DISACCHARIDES	Lactose	Specific dairy products, e.g. milk from animals
MONOSACCHARIDES	Excess fructose*	Specific fruit, juices, honey, high-fructose corn syrup, some flavoured waters
POLYOLS	Including mannitol and sorbitol	Specific fruit and vegetables Some low-calorie sweeteners, particularly those in sugar-free gums, mints and low-calorie products

* Remember: not all foods with fructose are restricted. As we discussed on page 118, many fruits contain enough glucose to help with the fructose absorption or, in the case of the theatre analogy, the glucose opens up that second viewing room.

How does it work?

As we touched on, unlike other carbohydrates (such as glucose), FODMAPs aren't completely absorbed in the small intestine and instead, they end up in the large intestine, which results in two things:

- **EXCESS FLUID:** The undigested carbohydrates (FODMAPs) can draw fluid from the body into the intestine, effectively dumping a load of extra fluid, increasing the pressure on the intestinal wall. This may also overwhelm the large intestine's ability to absorb the fluid, which can result in mushy, loose poops. Others may find that, although the start of their poop is hard and constipation-like (acting like a plug), the end of their poop may actually be loose.

- **FERMENTATION:** Yes, this is the GM food frenzy. As we touched on above, the FODMAPs entering the large intestine are rapidly eaten (more scientifically referred to as fermentation) by our GM. As a result, a burst of gas is released. Although this also occurs in people without IBS, in those with visceral hypersensitivity the stretching of the intestine activates the nerves around the intestine, triggering pain signals to the brain, as well as activating the tummy-distention reflex discussed on page 88.

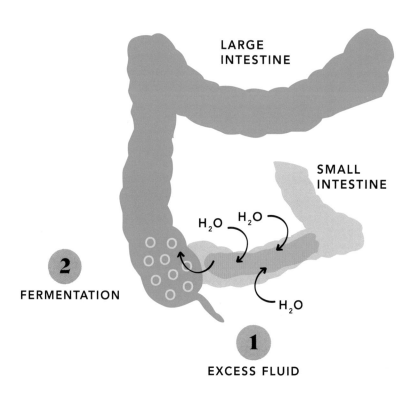

LARGE
INTESTINE

SMALL
INTESTINE

H_2O H_2O

2
FERMENTATION

H_2O

1

EXCESS FLUID

What does it involve?

A low-FODMAP diet consists of three stages, with the end goal being a personalized, modified FODMAP diet. You may read the stages below and feel slightly overwhelmed by the complexity of the diet and that's exactly why guidelines recommend that you embark on the low-FODMAP diet only with the support of a FODMAP-trained dietitian or health-care professional.

1

RESTRICTION STAGE: This is what people commonly refer to as the low-FODMAP diet, in that you restrict all high-FODMAP foods. It can help to think of this stage as giving your sensitive intestine some down time. Guidance from a dietitian is critical at this stage, in order to tailor the diet to your nutrient needs. If you don't respond to the diet after six weeks, revert to your usual diet and consider other therapies.

2

REINTRODUCTION STAGE: After following the restriction stage for two to six weeks (depending on how quickly your symptoms improve), you then reintroduce each of the different FODMAPs one at a time, in portions guided by your dietitian. This stage will help you identify which FODMAPs you're most sensitive to and the amount of offending FODMAPs you can tolerate without triggering symptoms. This stage can take several months to complete.

3

PERSONALIZATION STAGE: This is also known as the modified or personalized FODMAP diet (your long-term diet) and is the end product of Stages 1 and 2. This diet is tailored to your personal FODMAP tolerance. Stage 3 not only gives your diet flexibility and variation, a key factor in achieving long-term compliance, it keeps your GM happy and, above all, it improves your food-related quality of life. It's also worth keeping in mind that tolerance typically improves over time with the continuation of those gut–brain axis strategies, which we discuss in Chapter 7. For this reason, re-testing foods that you previously didn't tolerate is a good idea.

Principles worth knowing

- **A LOW-FODMAP DIET IS NOT FODMAP-FREE.** The diet categorizes food as 'high' or 'low' FODMAP, based on a cut-off level of FODMAPs per portion. This means that even low-FODMAP foods may contain some FODMAPs.

- **IT'S ALL ABOUT THE SIZE OF THE PORTION.** A high-FODMAP food may be low-FODMAP if the portion size is reduced. An example is wheat pasta. One cup of cooked wheat pasta is considered high FODMAP, whereas half a cup is considered low FODMAP.

- **LACTOSE IS A 'CONDITIONAL' FODMAP.** If you've gone through the 3R Method on page 122 and are confident that you're not lactose intolerant, then you don't need to restrict lactose in your low-FODMAP diet. With that in mind, even if you are lactose intolerant, you can still tolerate small amounts of lactose, as discussed on page 134. This is why the restriction stage allows some cow's milk (up to 50ml per sitting) and other dairy products that contain small amounts of lactose, such as hard cheeses (see page 129).

- **FODMAPS ARE CARBOHYDRATES.** It's helpful to remember that foods free of carbohydrates such as meats, seafood, egg, fats and oils are naturally free of FODMAPs (unless of course they've been marinated or use carbohydrate fillers/substitutes).

- **A LOW-FODMAP DIET IS NOT GLUTEN-FREE.** It is easy to get confused, because a low-FODMAP diet also restricts gluten-containing grains like wheat, barley and rye. The difference is that a low-FODMAP diet is restricting the large amounts of fructans found in these grains, rather than the gluten component. Therefore, the diet only restricts significant amounts of these grains, and lesser amounts can still be included, such as small amounts of wheat used in sauces. In contrast, a gluten-free diet restricts even trace amounts of these grains.

Mile-high IBS

Do your symptoms get worse on aeroplanes? There is some science behind this phenomenon. Air trapped inside your gut expands as the aeroplane climbs, thanks to the change in atmospheric pressure (this also explains why your ears pop and your water bottle or packets of food expand). Therefore, what might be only a little bit of gas at ground level can expand in the sky, putting extra pressure on your intestines. Although this happens with everyone, because those with IBS typically have a more sensitive intestine, this extra pressure can lead to feelings of bloating and pain. The solution? Cutting back on higher-FODMAP foods (see page 151) twenty-four to forty-eight hours before you fly may help.

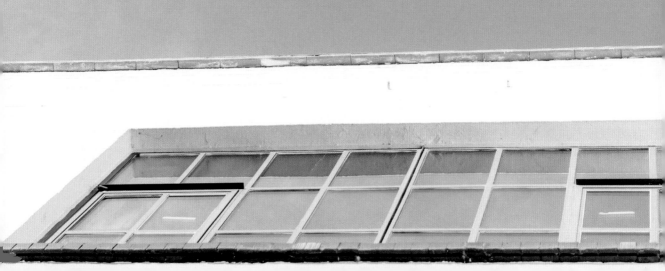

Real-world approach

I once tried to follow the low-FODMAP diet, not because I had IBS but because I wanted to experience it from my patients' perspective. I failed miserably! In the first week, I made a ton of mistakes; the second week, I ate the same meal four nights in a row because work was crazy busy and I hadn't planned ahead; and by the third week, I was craving my fudgy black bean brownies (see page 253) so badly that I pulled the plug. This experience taught me two things: first, my patients' symptoms must be pretty bad to be motivated enough to stick to the diet for up to six weeks; and second, the diet is really not forgiving of a lifestyle that is anything but ideal in terms of time and space to cook from scratch. This got me thinking: do all my patients really need to go the whole way to see benefits? It turns out that NO they don't – a simplified low-FODMAP diet, or 'FODMAP-lite' approach, restricting only a subset of high-FODMAP foods, is enough for many people with IBS to get control over their IBS.

Take, for example, twenty-one-year-old Toni. Toni had just moved out of home for university and was flat-sharing with five others. Having been diagnosed with IBS during her A-levels and trying first-line strategies with little benefit, Toni was keen to do whatever it took to get her symptoms under control before her university exams. However, it was clear that a low-FODMAP diet was not going to be appropriate with Toni's current lifestyle. In fact, it might have actually contributed to Toni's stress-induced symptoms due to the difficulty of following it .When I reviewed Toni's diet, I could see she was having large amounts of FODMAPs and was a good candidate for the FODMAP-lite approach (alongside mindfulness strategies). Within two weeks on the modified diet her symptoms had improved, and by week four she described her symptoms as 'completely under control'. Using the FODMAP-lite-approach, Toni was able to move swiftly through the next two stages. She identified her breakfast smoothie, large amounts of legumes, date-based energy balls and low-calorie sweets as her main triggers. To manage these, she turned her breakfast smoothie into whole foods – oats, fruit and yoghurt; reduced her portion of legumes at each sitting to her tolerated amount; and she started making her own energy balls minus the dates. As for the daily fifteen minutes of mindfulness, Toni found it had the added benefit of improving her concentration so she stuck with that long term.

If your IBS doesn't respond to the first-line diet approach and you don't have access to a FODMAP-trained health-care professional, the FODMAP-lite approach might be a helpful place to start. But don't just jump straight into it (the mistake I made with the full diet). Spend time becoming familiar with the higher-FODMAP foods and planning your meals without them. This will help you get the most out of the diet and minimize the burden and duration needed to follow the diet to see a benefit.

Select higher-FODMAP foods to limit	Examples of alternatives*
VEGETABLES Artichokes, asparagus, broccoli, Brussels sprouts, cabbage, cauliflower, chicory root, garlic, leeks, mushrooms, onions, spring onions (white part), peas.	Aubergines, carrots, chives, courgettes, cucumber, ginger, green beans, kale, peppers, potatoes, pumpkin, spinach, tomatoes, pickled garlic and onion.
FRUIT Apples, apricots, blackberries, boysenberries, cherries, dates, figs, mango, nectarines, peaches, pears, persimmons (Sharon fruit), plums, prunes, watermelon, fruit juice (more than 100ml), foods/drinks with added fruit concentrate.	Blueberries, clementines, honeydew melon, grapes, kiwis, lemons, limes, oranges, passion fruit, pineapple, raspberries, rhubarb, strawberries. Maximum of 1 piece of any fruit per sitting (equivalent of 80g fresh, 30g dried, 100ml juice), with a maximum of three sittings across the day.
PROTEIN SOURCES Legumes (e.g. baked beans, chickpeas, kidney beans, soya beans), pistachio nuts and cashews.	All fresh meats (e.g. chicken, fish, lamb), eggs, firm tofu, walnuts, Brazil nuts. Tinned and (thoroughly) rinsed legumes, contain fewer FODMAPs compared to those boiled from dry. Therefore, small portions (¼ cup per sitting), particularly of tinned chickpeas, butterbeans and adzuki beans, are better tolerated. ½ cup of tinned lentils is considered low-FODMAP.
GRAINS Keep to ½ cup of cooked or 1 slice of wheat, barley or rye-based foods per sitting (including couscous and semolina), with up to three across the day.	Quinoa, rice, buckwheat, millet, oats, polenta.
OTHER Agave, honey, high-fructose corn syrup, fructose and low-calorie sweeteners ending in -ol (see page 143). Added inulin, fructo-oligosaccharide, galacto-oligosaccharide in some yoghurts and cereals.	Golden syrup, maple syrup, table sugar (sucrose), glucose.

This is not a comprehensive list, instead it is to give you inspiration. Include all other foods that are not listed on the 'higher-FODMAP' column in your diet. Remember this is a modified version, not the full low-FODMAP diet.

FODMAP-lite approach

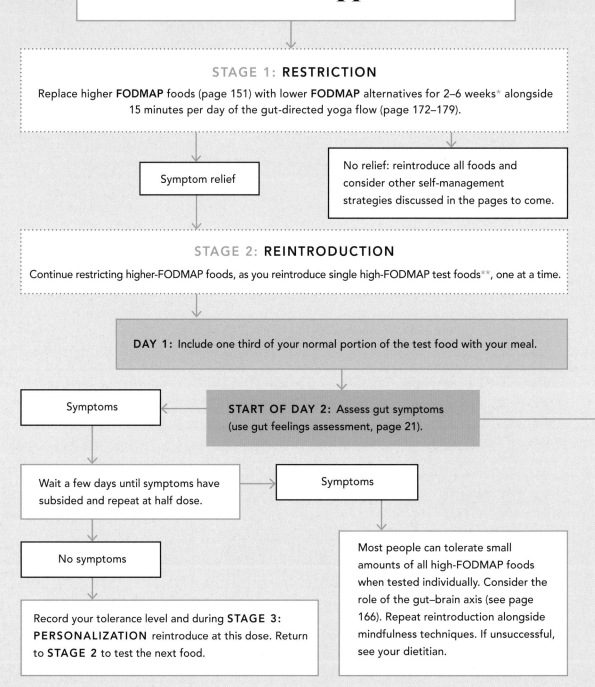

STAGE 1: RESTRICTION

Replace higher **FODMAP** foods (page 151) with lower **FODMAP** alternatives for 2–6 weeks* alongside 15 minutes per day of the gut-directed yoga flow (page 172–179).

Symptom relief

No relief: reintroduce all foods and consider other self-management strategies discussed in the pages to come.

STAGE 2: REINTRODUCTION

Continue restricting higher-FODMAP foods, as you reintroduce single high-FODMAP test foods**, one at a time.

DAY 1: Include one third of your normal portion of the test food with your meal.

Symptoms

START OF DAY 2: Assess gut symptoms (use gut feelings assessment, page 21).

Wait a few days until symptoms have subsided and repeat at half dose.

Symptoms

No symptoms

Record your tolerance level and during **STAGE 3: PERSONALIZATION** reintroduce at this dose. Return to **STAGE 2** to test the next food.

Most people can tolerate small amounts of all high-FODMAP foods when tested individually. Consider the role of the gut–brain axis (see page 166). Repeat reintroduction alongside mindfulness techniques. If unsuccessful, see your dietitian.

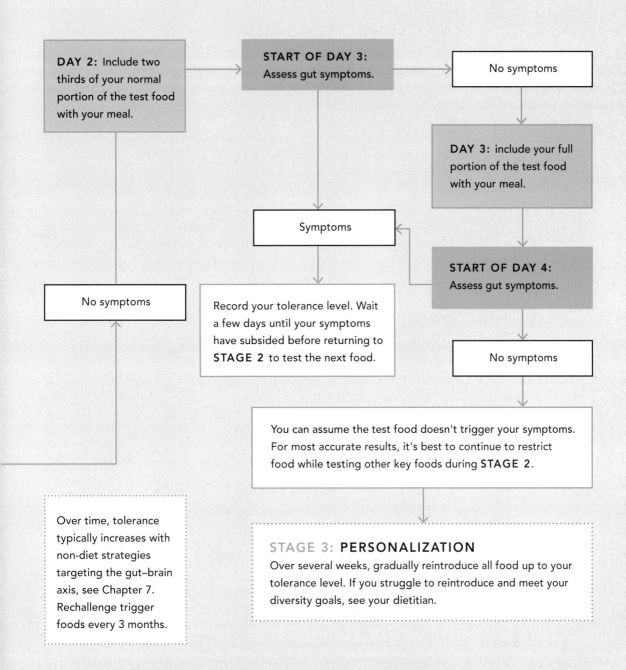

DAY 2: Include two thirds of your normal portion of the test food with your meal.

START OF DAY 3: Assess gut symptoms.

No symptoms

DAY 3: include your full portion of the test food with your meal.

Symptoms

No symptoms

Record your tolerance level. Wait a few days until your symptoms have subsided before returning to **STAGE 2** to test the next food.

START OF DAY 4: Assess gut symptoms.

No symptoms

You can assume the test food doesn't trigger your symptoms. For most accurate results, it's best to continue to restrict food while testing other key foods during **STAGE 2**.

Over time, tolerance typically increases with non-diet strategies targeting the gut–brain axis, see Chapter 7. Rechallenge trigger foods every 3 months.

STAGE 3: **PERSONALIZATION**
Over several weeks, gradually reintroduce all food up to your tolerance level. If you struggle to reintroduce and meet your diversity goals, see your dietitian.

* *Ensure you are maintaining adequate amounts of fruit, vegetables and wholegrains.*

** *TEST FOODS: Choose suspected trigger foods from higher FODMAP foods (page 151).*

Fibre supplements

Fibre in IBS can be a little confusing. Not only is the amount important – either too much or too little in your diet can trigger symptoms – but the type of fibre also matters. Rest assured, I won't bore you with all the intricacies; instead, let's focus on the most promising fibre supplement.

Psyllium (ispaghula)

This unique fibre has dual functionality, thickening up loose poops but at the same time softening hard poops. Therefore, it's thought to benefit all types of IBS by normalizing poop output. This may also improve other symptoms, such as bloating and incomplete evacuation. On its own, however, psyllium is unlikely to resolve all your IBS symptoms, so if you are interested in supplements, I recommend you use it in combination with other strategies.

PSYLLIUM PRESCRIPTION

Start with ½ tbsp/day (3g) and see how things go. You may like to increase to 1 tbsp/day in the second week if needed, gradually increasing up to 3 tbsp/day if useful and tolerated. If no improvement after one month, stop. If your gut is extra-sensitive, you may like to start with 1 teaspoon a day. The practical tips:

- *It's available from most health-food stores.*

- *It forms a thick gel when mixed with cold water (similar to what happens in your gut), so is best combined with porridge or warm soup. I often add to my granola too (see page 201). Have alongside 150ml of fluid/tbsp.*

- *Check in with your GP if needing to take for over 6 months.*

- *Like many fibres, psyllium can decrease your appetite. If you are underweight, it may be best to stick to the half-dose and continue to monitor your weight. If your weight decreases, stop and discuss with your dietitian.*

Flaxseed

In terms of food sources, there is some evidence for flaxseed in constipation-predominant IBS (IBS-C). If you want to give it a go, I recommend that you start with half a tablespoon a day (6g) and gradually increase up to 2 tablespoons a day over four weeks, as needed and tolerated. Sprinkle some on your breakfast, yoghurt, salads or soups. Be sure to include an extra 150ml fluid/1 tbsp of flaxseeds. Check out the high-flaxseed crackers on page 245.

Peppermint oil

Unlike many other herbal supplements, the benefits of peppermint oil in IBS have been rigorously studied and are backed by quality science (and a heap of anecdotes from my patients, too). Peppermint oil is an anti-spasmodic, which means it works by relaxing a tense intestine, something that's common in IBS. As a result, peppermint oil has been shown to significantly reduce tummy pain. It may also help relieve tummy bloating and excess wind by supporting more efficient gas transport.

What about peppermint tea? The studies showing the benefits of peppermint oil have only used coated peppermint-oil capsules. Why does the coating matter? It stops the oil being digested in the stomach, ensuring it make its way into the small intestine, where the peppermint works its magic. That's not to say that drinking peppermint tea is pointless: if you find it helps, then do what works for you.

The practical stuff

If you're interested in giving peppermint oil a try, studies recommend taking one capsule (providing 0.2ml or 180–225mg of peppermint oil) up to three times a day, thirty minutes to an hour before a meal. It's generally best to take on an empty stomach and away from antacids. Most studies have used specific peppermint-oil products (Colpermin or Mintoil), which are widely available from health stores or online. In terms of safety (because anything in a high dose is always worth checking), peppermint capsules have been shown to be well tolerated, but long-term studies have not been done. Given this, you might like to consider tapering down after four weeks, and anything beyond two months is worth discussing with your healthcare team.

Managing stubborn tummy pain

If diet and supplements don't relieve your tummy pain, as well as natural remedies like applying a heat pack to the painful site, talk to your GP about medications that can help. These include anti-spasmodics such as hyoscine butylbromide (e.g. Buscopan), which can be handy to keep in your bag if you're prone to unpredictable IBS-related cramping episodes. For long-term pain, there are a group of medications known as central neuromodulators that have proven effective via targeting the gut–brain pain pathway. Interestingly, these central modulators are a type of antidepressant, although for IBS are prescribed at much lower doses.

Small intestinal bacterial overgrowth

Commonly referred to as SIBO, small intestinal bacterial overgrowth is characterized by an increased number of microbes invading the small intestine. The small intestine is much more sensitive than the large intestine and so it doesn't fare well when having to accommodate these extra microbial guests (and their fermenting feasts). As a consequence, they can interfere with the small intestine's normal functioning, causing IBS-like symptoms such as tummy pain, bloating, excess flatulence and diarrhoea.

It's still early days in terms of our understanding of SIBO, but it is thought that it may overlap or account for a subset of IBS. Breath tests are commonly used in practice to support diagnosis. However, there are considerable limitations with breath tests, and therefore interpretation of results should be guided by a specialist gut doctor (gastroenterologist), or trained health-care professional.

Disappointingly, there is limited research into the dietary management of SIBO, although a low-FODMAP diet is likely to reduce gut symptoms. This is because the diet decreases the amount of fermentable food available in the lower end of the small intestine where the overgrowth occurs, essentially starving the overgrown microbe community. The standard therapy for SIBO is antibiotic treatment. Research suggests that combining the antibiotic with a special fibre known as hydrolysed guar gum, which you can buy online or from health-food stores, may have a greater benefit compared to using the antibiotic alone (one study showed an 85 per cent success rate with the combination, compared to 62 per cent with antibiotics alone). Another study demonstrated that combining the antibiotic with a probiotic also enhanced the effectiveness. Nonetheless, it is worth keeping in mind that the relapse rates post antibiotic are disappointingly high. This is because antibiotics are only treating the symptoms and not the underlying cause of the overgrowth. It's worth discussing with your gut doctor ways to prevent relapse of SIBO.

One for the ladies

As some of you will know all too well, IBS symptoms can get worse leading up to and/or during menstruation. This is related to fluctuating hormones that not only affect your uterus but also target your gut, affecting motility, sensitivity and levels of inflammation. If your periods are particularly painful or heavy, however, it's worth visiting your GP to be assessed for endometriosis, a condition that affects as many as one in ten women. Despite many overlaps with IBS, some of the red flags for endometriosis include difficulty conceiving, painful sex and heavy periods.

Maybe it's not IBS

If you've got diarrhoea-predominant IBS (IBS-D) (not sure of your type? Go to the assessment on page 139), it's worth paying particular attention to whether your symptoms are worse after high-fat meals. If you see a pattern and notice that your diarrhoea improves to some extent on a low-fat diet, it's worth discussing the possibility of bile acid diarrhoea (BAD) with your GP. Why? As we touched on on page 16, bile acids are released to help our body absorb fat and, while 95 per cent is normally reabsorbed in the small intestine, in some cases it's not and instead it enters the large intestine, causing havoc and resulting in diarrhoea. Research suggests that as many as 30 per cent of people with IBS-D may actually have BAD, which means that it's the malabsorption of the bile acids in the intestine that's causing the diarrhoea, not IBS. If this is the case, there are different management strategies, including both medication and dietary approaches, that are best discussed with your GP and dietitian, respectively.

When self-management is not enough

If your symptoms are still getting the better of you after trying the strategies detailed in this chapter, it's time to call in the gut experts. I know this can be frustrating, but remember, we've only touched on the basics here; there are plenty of other strategies your GP, dietitian and gastroenterologist have up their sleeves. If you're feeling alone on your journey, most countries have an IBS charity which includes IBS support groups that are worth tapping into – they have been life-changing for many of my patients. (Check out www.theibsnetwork.org.)

CHAPTER 7

Beyond diet:
sleep, stress and exercise

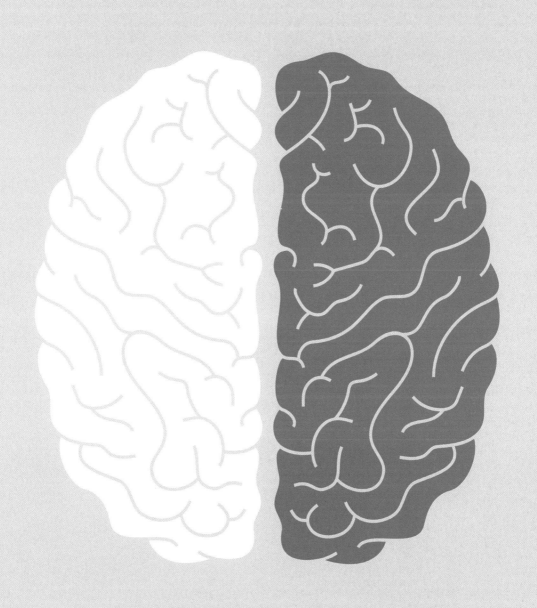

Beyond diet

Let's explore what else you can do to take your budding relationship with your gut to the next level. Outside of diet, there are three areas I see as being key for good gut health: sleep, stress and exercise. Their importance for overall health is clearly nothing new, but what is new is our understanding of how they impact our gut microbiota (GM). If we really want to harness the full potential of our gut health, we also need to get these three main areas in check.

Advice around 'sleeping more' and 'stressing less' has become redundant: we all know we should be doing it, yet too few of us are. Life happens – I totally get it. This is why I want to share with you the tools, the exercises and the strategies, and help you fit them in around everything else going on in your life. For those of you who are thinking, I don't have time for this, I'm just going to stick with diet, I hear you, but here's the thing: you can have the 'ultimate' gut-boosting diet, but if you're not sleeping right or your stress levels are through the roof, your gut health will likely pay the price. Just as they say that no amount of exercise can outdo a bad diet, no amount of gut-boosting eating can outdo a disastrous lifestyle. Balance really is the key to your GM's heart.

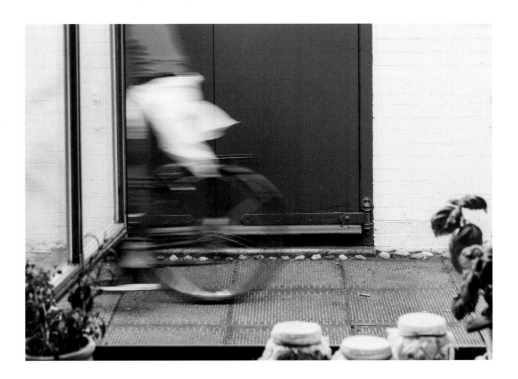

One of my patients, forty-three-year-old Emma, experienced first hand the importance of balance. Emma was a single mum, juggling bringing up two young kids with full-time work. She was considered quite the superwoman among her friends.

Over two months we worked together to get Emma to a place where she had good control of her symptoms through diet, apart from the occasional episode. After some troubleshooting of various potential causes we identified poor sleep and stress as two of her key triggers. To target these areas, Emma and I developed a fifteen-minute programme of strategies (many of which are covered in this chapter) as a preventative measure, to help Emma cope when these unavoidable circumstances arose. Three months later, when I saw her again, I could tell from the look on her face that something had happened. Emma recounted her worst episode yet. She'd been at work when the tummy pain began, and within an hour it had become so crippling that she'd had to swallow her pride and ask her colleague to take her to the emergency department and her neighbour to collect her kids from school.

How had this happened? Emma explained that she'd had a very hectic month and, between a promotion at work and looking after the kids, her fifteen-minute programme had dropped off her schedule. Reflecting back, it was clear to her that by not allowing herself those fifteen minutes each day, it ended up costing her over three days in down time (that's over 2,000 minutes!) at the expense of both her family and work.

Emma's case is an extreme example of how not taking a few moments out each day to look after yourself could end up costing you much more in the long run. I think there is something we can all learn from Emma's experience: are you taking at least fifteen minutes a day to focus on your health and happiness?

For each of these non-diet 'heavy hitters', we'll go through a range of practical strategies and exercises that I've seen first hand make a meaningful impact on people's lives. It's a good idea to record the ones that resonated with you in your gut-health action plan on page 282. Throughout this chapter, keep in mind that anything is better than nothing. Even if you only manage to add in a small change, you'll still be one step ahead of where you were yesterday.

Sleep

One of the most underrated resources at your disposal to support optimal (gut) health is sleep. Like our human cells, our GM has a circadian rhythm (a body clock), so disturbed sleep can also impact its natural rhythm, as we touched on in Chapter 2. Studies have shown that sleep deprivation can impact our GM after just two days of getting less sleep than we need. Sleep deprivation can also increase inflammation and stress hormones in your body, which may explain why not getting enough sleep is linked with worse gut symptoms, particularly in people with irritable bowel syndrome (IBS).

Work by my colleagues at King's College London has shown that lack of sleep can also impact how much you eat. And it's not by a nominal amount either – the review study suggested that partial sleep deprivation increased daily intake by the calorie equivalent of four slices of bread. As you may have experienced yourself – I know I have – this extra food tended not to be the quality high-fibre stuff: the study showed that sleep-deprived people grabbed for more of the high-fat, lower-protein foods, keeping all the nutrition to themselves and leaving none for their poor GM (who, don't forget, have also been sleep-deprived).

When you haven't had enough sleep, you are also more susceptible to getting sick. One study which used identical twins to control for genetics found that sleep deprivation was linked with lower immunity (remember: 70 per cent of our immune cells live in the gut).

Before we move on to looking at the practical strategies to help boost your pillow time, it's worth thinking about your sleep quality. How refreshed do you feel most days?

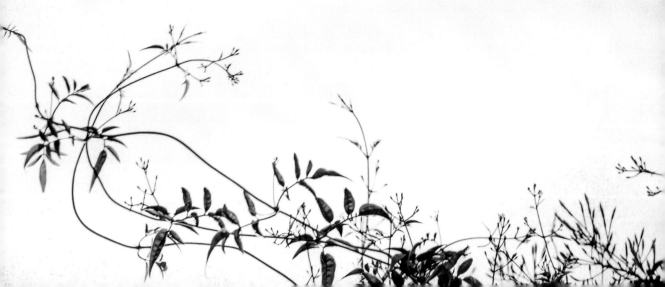

Assessment : SLEEP QUALITY AND IMMUNITY

The first assessment relates to your usual sleep habits. I know sleeping habits are not always the same, but try to think about your average sleep when completing this assessment. What about your immune system? Are you frequently catching the flu, or do you struggle to shake an infection? Head over to www.TheGutHealthDoctor.com to complete the sleep-quality and immunity assessments.

One in three adults don't get enough good-quality sleep – how did yours rate? If your sleep quality is on the lower end, rest assured, it's certainly not a life sentence. Improving your sleep can be achieved by making small changes to your lifestyle. Colleagues Dr Al Khatib and Dr Hall proved this in a trial where, using simple sleep-hygiene strategies, they were able to significantly improve not just sleep duration but participants' sleep quality, too. They also showed the knock-on benefit of improved sleep on diet. In fact, compared to the control group (who maintained their usual sleeping pattern), those who applied the sleep strategies reduced their intake of added sugars by two teaspoons per day – which is pretty impressive, given that diet wasn't the focus.

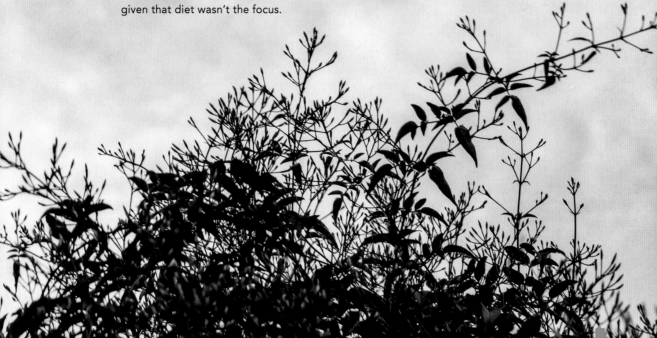

Dr Al Khatib and colleagues' Sleep Hygiene Protocol

First up, what does 'sleep hygiene' actually mean? It's a buzz phrase that describes the habits you can put in place to optimize the length and quality of your sleep. The result? You feel much better rested and begin to reap the knock-on effects, including benefits to your immunity, diet and other areas of your well-being, such as mood.

STEP 1: *Identify four habits from the sleep-hygiene checklist that are relevant and realistic targets for your lifestyle.*

STEP 2: *Implement your chosen strategies for a minimum of four weeks.*

STEP 3: *After four weeks, reassess your sleep quality using the sleep-quality assessment.*

STEP 4: *Re-evaluate your selected strategies and adjust as needed, keeping in mind that it typically takes nine weeks of daily practice to form a habit (or sixty-six days, to be exact, according to research from University College London). If you have persistent sleeplessness, it's worth speaking to your GP or a sleep expert for support.*

SLEEP-HYGIENE CHECKLIST:

1. A REGULAR ROUTINE: Maintaining the same sleep time and wake time every day (give or take 30 minutes) can help your body's and GM's clock to function at their best.

2. BEDROOM ENVIRONMENT: Make your bedroom a relaxing environment that you use only for sleep (and bonding with your partner). To do this, keep your bedroom:

   • **Dark:** make sure you keep your bedroom only dimly lit at night by using dimmers or lamps with low-wattage bulbs. It also may be worth investing in some thick curtains (or an eye mask).

   • **Tidy and quiet:** clutter and noise can distract your mind from relaxing. Try some earplugs, if you need them.

- **At a slightly cool temperature** (around 18°C): your body's temperature starts to drop as you fall deeper into your slumber, and so it helps not to get too warm while you sleep.

3. MORNING LIGHT: Light is how your environment communicates with your body clock. Exposing your face to natural light first thing in the morning helps support and reset your body clock. Whether it's going for a five-minute walk outside, or doing some stretching in your backyard, waking your body with natural light is a really refreshing way to start your day.

4. TECHNOLOGY (including TVs, laptops, phones and other gadgets): Blue light from back-lit screens is particularly disruptive to your body's clock. It counteracts your ability to produce melatonin, which is an important hormone for sleep. Avoid these in the hours before bedtime. If you must use them, consider installing 'blue light filter' apps on your device.

5. NAPPING: Avoid excessive napping during the day (more than twenty minutes). You may not feel tired enough to fall asleep at night.

6. AVOID CAFFEINE AND STIMULANTS: These oppose your body's attempts to wind down before bedtime and it's best to limit them after 3 p.m.

7. FULLNESS/HUNGER: Going to bed too full or hungry can disrupt your sleep. Depending on the size of your meal, waiting at least two to three hours before bed can be helpful. Similarly, if you are too hungry, you may be too distracted to fall asleep and may wake up through the night wanting a snack.

8. A BEDTIME ROUTINE TO HELP YOU UNWIND:
- Have a warm bath (not too hot) to relax you and help your body reach a temperature that is ideal for rest.

- Relaxation exercises such as gentle stretching can help your muscles to relax.

- Listen to music that calms you, or even a guided smartphone meditation app to help calm your thoughts.

- Reading a book in dim light is a great alternative to being on your phone or laptop in the bedroom.

9. SCHEDULE 'WORRY TIME': We often struggle to fall asleep if we're worrying. It may sound counter-intuitive but allowing yourself some time during your day to 'worry' and write down all your thoughts and to-do lists can give you the mental space to relax before bed.

Stress: rewiring the gut–brain axis

It's easy to get caught up in trying to 'perfect' your diet and forget that our brain has a big impact on our gut, too. If you're a little sceptical, as I first was, let me share the research with you. Several trials have compared, head to head, the effectiveness of the standard diet for IBS, a low-FODMAP diet (page 145) and non-diet approaches that target the gut–brain axis. The non-diet approaches included cognitive behavioural therapy (CBT), relaxation techniques, hypnotherapy and yoga. Strikingly, several trials showed that the non-diet interventions improved gut symptoms to the same degree as the dietary intervention. Just think about that for a moment: one intervention solely targeting trigger foods and the other just the gut–brain axis, both with the same outcome. (It's worth noting that the non-diet approaches do take a little longer to take effect, so stick with them for at least 12 weeks.)

Rather than removing foods that can trigger the gut, the non-diet approaches work on the underlying cause, that is, the dysfunction between the gut and brain via the vagus nerve. The vagus nerve is the part of the nervous system that we likened to a mobile phone in Chapter 2, acting as a communication highway that connects our brain and our gut (and almost every other organ in between). This nerve plays a crucial role in breathing, in our heart rate, immune response and digestion. It's also part of the parasympathetic system (PNS, the rest-and-digest control centre), which, when activated, has a knock-on effect of settling the sympathetic system (SNS, the fight-or-flight control centre).

I used to rely on two ways to assess the impact of the gut–brain axis on my patients' symptoms. First, I'd ask them to rate their general day-to-day stress levels, and second, I'd get them to consider whether their symptoms improved when they were on holiday. From this quick assessment I would determine how much of a priority it was to focus on stress… but after meeting twenty-four-year-old Kelly I realized assessing stress was not that straightforward. Kelly had been diagnosed with IBS and had been referred by her gastroenterologist for dietary advice. I went through my standard assessment and stress didn't flag up; she had a below-average score and no change to gut symptoms on holidays. Kelly appeared to be a good candidate for the low-FODMAP diet. At our follow-up review, as I'd expected, Kelly's symptoms had resolved, but what I didn't expect was the way it had come about. Hint: diet had nothing to do with it.

Kelly had been following the low-FODMAP diet for two weeks before she went away to a friend's wedding. At that stage, Kelly hadn't noticed much improvement in her symptoms but was committed to following the diet for at least four weeks, despite the challenges of doing so while on holiday. Within a few days of being away, she noticed her symptoms were starting to improve, despite not being as strict with the diet as she'd intended. By day five, Kelly described herself as feeling like a new woman; after years of battling with her symptoms, it seemed they had disappeared. The eczema across her chest had also started to clear. A few days later, Kelly returned from the wedding and continued to follow the diet. Within days, her symptoms had returned with a vengeance. 'As defeating as it was,' she said, 'I'm glad it happened. It was the wake-up call I needed to realize I was unconsciously battling stress.'

Kelly had an easy-going boss, a loving partner, no money issues – she felt she didn't have the right to be stressed, so suppressed any feelings of it. Like many of us, Kelly always jam-packed her holidays with activities and never really switched off for more than a day. 'This time,' Kelly reflected, 'every element was organized for me. I just had to turn up. I slept in most days and lay by the pool. There was bad internet, so I didn't bother with my phone – it was the first time in years that I'd truly disconnected.'

With this new level of awareness, Kelly had begun to see a psychologist and, within three weeks of therapy, was starting to get that new-woman vibe back. Diet-wise, we reintroduced all high-FODMAP foods and moved towards the gut health on a plate principles (pages 70–71).

Kelly's story is a familiar one. Modern life is so busy that many of us underestimate how stressed we really are. In fact, in many cultures, being stressed has become the new norm and being busy a badge of honour. While we may be used to it, the signs of this unconscious stress often present through other ways such as troubled sleep, unstable mood and gut issues.

Assessment: IS STRESS GETTING THE BETTER OF YOU?

Although it's normal and often beneficial for everyone to get a little stressed from time to time, if it is frequent or debilitating when it does strike, your (gut) health is likely paying the price. Even if you don't think you're stressed, it's worth checking. Head over to www.TheGutHealthDoctor.com to complete the stress assessment.

The strategies

Many of us, including myself, have at some stage fallen for the idea that it is good to be constantly on the go. But our brains and bodies are not made to be relentlessly on the go; they become fatigued and this raises stress levels, decreases resilience and impacts our GM. Rest is as important as activity for our physical, mental and gut health. Gut-brain expert psychologist Kimberly Wilson recommends two of her favourite exercises to help target your gut–brain axis that you can try out in the comfort of your own home.

• EXERCISE 1: the do-nothing exercise

This exercise is essentially scheduled inactivity. Many stressed people find this one really challenging, as we can worry about being unproductive or 'lazy'. Sometimes, underlying this is a feeling that, if we stop, we won't have the energy to start again. This is a good clue to how tired and stressed we really feel.

'Do nothing' is exactly that. You need to decide a point in the day where you do absolutely nothing. Ideally, it's best to lie down so that there isn't even any physical stimulation. With that in mind, many people find it best to do this at the end of the working day, when you get home. It is particularly useful before having a meal.

Place a notepad and pen beside you (you won't need them until the end). Set a timer for ten minutes (if using your phone be sure to switch to silent). Lie down on your back; you can have your knees up or down, whichever is more comfortable. Rest your hands on your tummy or by your side. Take one or two deep breaths to settle yourself and then just notice what happens. Consider the questions opposite. Try to stay with these experiences and, at the end of the ten minutes, write down your observations.

This exercise can give you a really good insight into your attitudes towards yourself. Is it good to be busy? Do you imagine that someone else seeing you have a rest would call you lazy? Seeing these ideas written down in black and white can help you to challenge them in exercise 2.

Try this exercise once in the first week and slowly build up to at least five times a week, particularly on your busiest days.

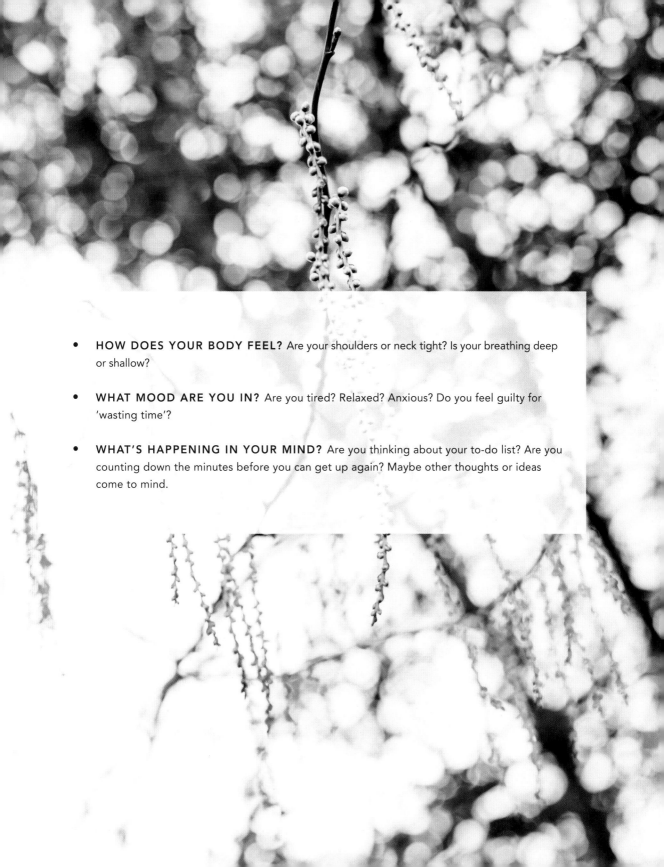

- **HOW DOES YOUR BODY FEEL?** Are your shoulders or neck tight? Is your breathing deep or shallow?

- **WHAT MOOD ARE YOU IN?** Are you tired? Relaxed? Anxious? Do you feel guilty for 'wasting time'?

- **WHAT'S HAPPENING IN YOUR MIND?** Are you thinking about your to-do list? Are you counting down the minutes before you can get up again? Maybe other thoughts or ideas come to mind.

• **EXERCISE 2:**
challenging judgemental thoughts (CBT)

The do-nothing exercise often throws light on our unconscious mental habits. Typically, we hold ourselves to much higher standards than we do others. We are much more critical of ourselves than we would be of a friend, or even a stranger, in the same situation. This constant internal pressure (as well as external demands) is a major driver of stress and poor coping. Recognizing and managing stress is dependent on our ability to be compassionate to ourselves, to treat ourselves like we would our best friend. I know it can be an odd concept for many, but trust me: it's worth thinking about.

One way to start challenging judgemental thoughts about ourselves is to imagine you are hearing your own story from someone else. If a friend told you they were pushing themselves non-stop and never giving themselves a break, what would you say? Would you tell them to just suck it up, that they should be able to keep up with the pace, or would you say, 'Wow, it sounds like you're under a lot of pressure'? Would you be curious about why they were being so hard on themselves? Write down the kinder and more balanced things you would say to a friend. Then, when those critical, pressurizing thoughts come up, try directing those more supportive thoughts to yourself. It's important to begin with something that feels manageable, so start by challenging just one critical thought that you have experienced. Once that positive challenge becomes automatic, you can move on to another critical thought.

Sometimes, critical thoughts and beliefs are deeply entrenched and it can be helpful to see a psychologist who can help support you in understanding where those thoughts may have come from and how to challenge them.

Depending on how you scored on the stress assessment, it might be a good idea to try to stick to at least one of these exercises for twelve weeks. I know sticking with things is easier said than done. To help, check out my top habit-forming tips on page 288.

Yoga

Yoga is a practice of the mind–body (and, I'm convinced, GM too) that originated thousands of years ago. Coming from a science background, for a long time I thought yoga was a little too hippie-dippie for me. However, after putting my preconceived judgements aside and experiencing it for myself, I realized that not only did it improve my own focus, but it was underpinned by several scientific principles. In fact, a systematic review (remember: that's the collection of evidence from multiple trials) has suggested that yoga practice may actually decrease inflammation markers in our blood, meaning there are tangible benefits of yoga on our whole body. Another review has shown benefits in people with high blood pressure. I've got some anecdotes from my clinic, too, where several patients have had their GP reduce (and some even stop) their blood-pressure medication after three months of practising a daily yoga flow including the breathing exercise similar to that overleaf. In terms of gut disorders, it has been a game-changer for the long-term management of many of my patients too.

Yoga can relax a distressed gut in several ways. Not only does the breathing activate the PNS, that 'rest and digest' system, it teaches you how to embrace new and often uncomfortable feelings in your body through improved control of your breathing as you explore various positions. This valuable technique can be applied to episodes of tummy pain or other gut symptoms, breathing through the discomfort as you would through a yoga pose rather than resisting it, which creates greater anxiety and stress. The physical movements flowing between gentle compression and stretching also sends pulses along your intestine. This can help calm overall stimulation of the muscles and nerves and release any trapped gas (so if you get the urge let it out!) And the cherry on the top: most yoga sequences also end with relaxation, which you can think of as 'resetting' the gut–brain axis.

As we touched on, one trial found that yoga had equal benefits to a low-FODMAP diet, with over 80 per cent reporting significant improvement in their IBS symptoms. This research sparked my partnership with yoga teacher Richie Norton to develop a yoga sequence specifically for people with gut distress. Inspired by the postures used in the trial, we've developed a fifteen-minute sequence to make it a manageable daily addition to your morning or evening routine. Try it out and, for real results, stick with it for at least twelve weeks as they did in the trial.

Gut-directed yoga flow

The flow consists of four parts, all equally important: the warm-up, the breath, the moves and the calm. All help manage the physical and psychological symptoms of stress. If you suffer with IBS-related tummy pain, many of my patients have found implementing this practice, as soon as they feel an episode coming on, hugely beneficial in preventing the symptoms from escalating.

The warm-up

1. **FIND SOMEWHERE QUIET WHERE YOU CAN SIT WITHOUT BEING DISTURBED.** You can sit on the floor, on a cushion or on a chair, wherever you feel most comfortable sitting upright with a straight back to prevent squashing your belly.

2. **START TO BRING AWARENESS TO YOUR BREATHING,** taking deep breaths in through your nose then pausing for a few moments before gently releasing with a long, slow exhale, again through the nose. As you breathe in, feel the coolness of the air in your nostrils and its warmth as you breathe out.

3. **ONCE YOU'VE FOUND A STEADY, CALMING BREATHING RHYTHM,** begin to slowly loosen and mobilize the neck, shoulders and back with some gentle rolling movements, being mindful not to rush this.

 Caution: If you have issues with low or fluctuating blood pressure, it's best to discuss the breathing exercises with your GP first.

The breath

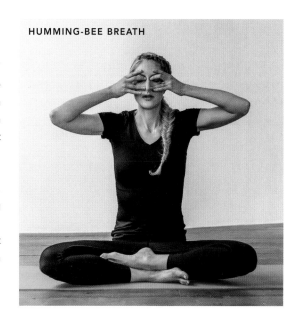

1. Sitting upright, connect to a deeper 'belly breath' (see below), making the inhale full and the exhale relaxed for ten breaths. If you've got some extra time on your hands, give the 'humming-bee breath' a try. Each style of breathing can relax you in different ways, so you might like to alternate between them.

2. If you are new to yoga and these breathing practices, it may feel more comfortable to start off by breathing in through your nose and out through your mouth. Over time, you can move to breathing in and out through your nose and see whether it makes a difference to how calm you feel.

Belly breath (diaphragmatic breathing)

1. Place one hand on your chest and one on your belly. Start by taking a relaxed, deep breath in through your nose. Take a note of which hand moves more, before gently releasing the air out through your nose (or mouth, if you prefer).

2. With your next breath in, allow your belly and rib cage to expand out, feeling your bottom hand rise while the hand on your chest remains still. This is a diaphragmatic breath. When you do this in reverse and the hand on your chest moves more, you are chest breathing. Chest breathing is designed for great exertion, which we subconsciously tend to activate in stressful situations. Making a conscious note to switch to diaphragmatic breathing in these situations can have a powerful calming effect.

Humming-bee breath (bhramari pranayama)

1. Sitting upright, with your eyes closed, raise your elbows to shoulder height and close your ears with your thumbs. Place your index finger above each eyebrow. Cover your eyelids with the middle fingers and place your ring finger beside the flare of each nostril (as pictured above).

2. Take a slow, deep breath to fill your lungs. Partially close your nostrils and breathe out through your nose, making a humming sound. Continue the humming for four seconds. Repeat five to ten times, extending the humming duration as you feel more comfortable with it.*

This is a great tool to use when you feel stress arise during the day. Whether it's a missed train, bad emails or lost keys . . . it's a game-changer.

The moves (asanas)

For those new to yoga, stick with the foundation flow detailed below. If you're more experienced, you may like to add in the advanced positions signposted with a double asterisk (**) to extend your flow. Hold each pose for at least three slow breaths.

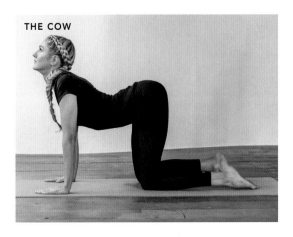

THE COW

Cat–Cow

Move on to all fours with your shoulders stacked over your hands and your knees positioned below your hips. Begin with some light movements side to side, forwards and backwards.

- **The cow:**

    Inhale, tilting your tailbone up, lifting your head and opening the chest, gazing slightly upwards. Be careful not to compress your neck.

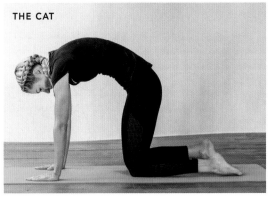

THE CAT

- **The cat:**

    With your exhale, tilt your chin to the chest, push away from the ground, opening your shoulders and back. (Tip: Visualize pulling your belly button into your spine.)

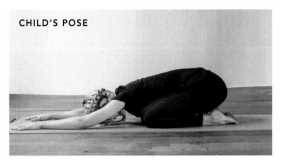

CHILD'S POSE

Child's pose

Return to your deep breaths (in and out through your nose), open out the knees and hips and ease yourself back, pushing from the hands until you are sitting over your heels. Let your forehead gently rest on the ground, letting your arms settle comfortably in front of you. Rest and breathe into the belly.

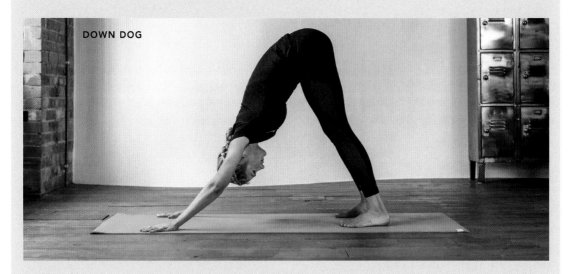

DOWN DOG

Optional: Down dog**

Move back on to all fours. Rolling your toes under, lift your knees off the ground, pushing your chest back towards your thighs. Try straightening your legs as much as your flexibility will allow and push your heels down to the ground (don't worry if they don't touch). Breathe through the gentle stretch that radiates along the back of your legs, continuing to move your chest towards your thighs, maximizing the stretch across the back of your shoulders.

Optional: Forward fold**

From down dog, walk your hands back towards your feet. Let your shoulders hang heavy over your feet. Slide your hands up along your legs, slowly bringing your chest parallel with the floor. Hold for one breath before moving to a full standing position, extending your arms wide, then drawing them in to meet above your head. Slowly lower your hands down the centre of your body, resting them in front of your chest bone in the prayer position.

Inhale, folding forward back into down dog.

Half-cobra

Lay yourself out flat on your front with your forearms flat and your hands in line with your shoulders. Take a breath in, and on the exhale gently push away from the floor, keeping contact along the arms. (Tip: Engage your leg muscles and lightly contract your glutes, i.e. your butt muscles.) Open up the front of your chest and belly. Relax back down and repeat.

HALF-COBRA

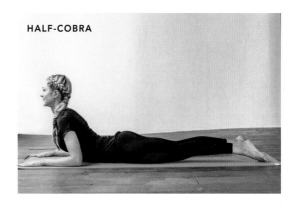

Optional: Locust pose**

Lie yourself flat on your front with your arms down by your side, palms planted on the floor. Gently contract your lower-back muscles and raise your chest and arms. Hold for two breaths before relaxing back down. Next, contract your glutes and lift your legs off the ground, pushing your pelvic bone into the floor. Relax down. Combine both movements together, as below.

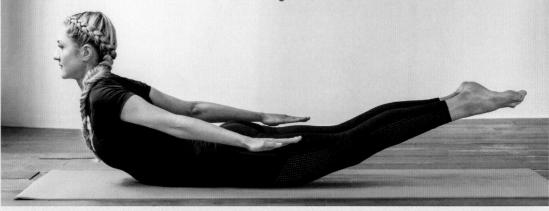

PIGEON POSE

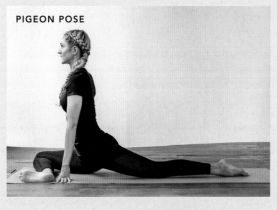

SAGE TWIST

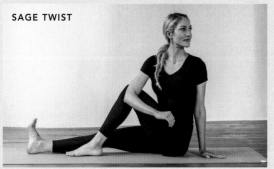

Optional: Pigeon pose**

Bring your right leg forward in between your hands and rest your knee next to your right hand and your foot towards your left hand (depending on your flexibility, your knee may be at anywhere from a 15- to a 90-degree angle). Gently lower your body weight evenly into both hips, keeping them straight, and extend your right leg back.

As you inhale, lengthen through the upper body and, as you exhale, sink a little deeper into your hips, pressing your right leg back into the floor and evening out the hips. Repeat on the other side.

Sage twist

Sit upright with your legs extended in front of you. Bend your left knee and hug it towards your chest. Place your left hand behind you for support as your right elbow moves to your left knee, lightly twisting the body. Repeat the twist on the other side.

Crocodile twist

Lying on your back, tuck both knees into your chest and gently rock side to side and back and forth, lightly massaging your back. Release the legs down before bringing your right leg across your body. Look to your opposite shoulder, hold and breathe. Repeat on the other side.

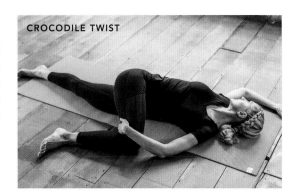

CROCODILE TWIST

Happy baby

Inhale bringing both knees into your chest. Bring your arms through the insides of your knees and hold on to the outside edge of each foot. Gently pull your knees down towards your underarms. Visualize pressing your tailbone down into the floor as you press your heels up, keeping them flat, as if you were standing on the ceiling. Press the shoulders and the back of your neck down into the floor, aiming to flatten your whole spine. Rock across your back, left to right. Smile like a happy baby.

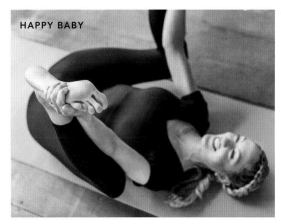

HAPPY BABY

Bridge pose

Lying on your back with your knees bent, push off the floor with your feet, lifting the hips, tightening your glutes to support your back and keeping your chin tucked into your chest. Breathe.

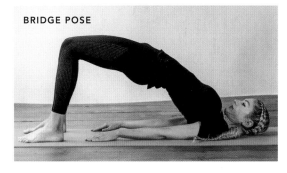

BRIDGE POSE

Corpse pose

Lower your back flat on the floor, bring your knees to your chest and rock side to side, forward and back. Then lay your legs out straight, allowing your feet to fall out to the side (open hips). Close your eyes, be still and breathe.

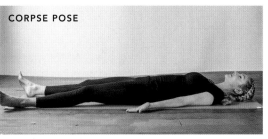

CORPSE POSE

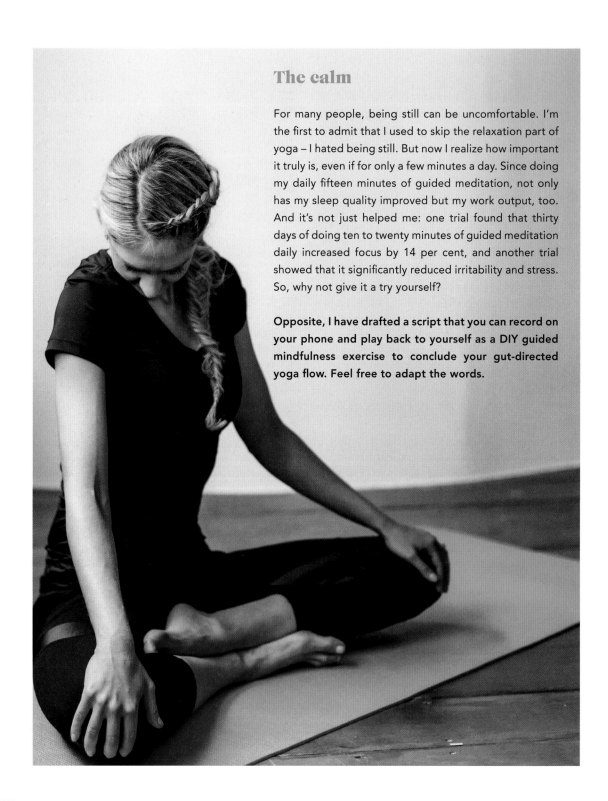

The calm

For many people, being still can be uncomfortable. I'm the first to admit that I used to skip the relaxation part of yoga – I hated being still. But now I realize how important it truly is, even if for only a few minutes a day. Since doing my daily fifteen minutes of guided meditation, not only has my sleep quality improved but my work output, too. And it's not just helped me: one trial found that thirty days of doing ten to twenty minutes of guided meditation daily increased focus by 14 per cent, and another trial showed that it significantly reduced irritability and stress. So, why not give it a try yourself?

Opposite, I have drafted a script that you can record on your phone and play back to yourself as a DIY guided mindfulness exercise to conclude your gut-directed yoga flow. Feel free to adapt the words.

The script

- **TAKE A FEW MOMENTS TO GET COMFORTABLE,** *whether it's staying in the corpse pose or sitting up with a straight back, cross-legged. Gently close your eyes. Begin by bringing your attention into a deep, slow belly breath, in through your nose and out freely through your mouth. Repeat for five breaths.*

- **BEGIN TO MOVE YOUR FOCUS INTO THE REST OF YOUR BODY.** *Feel the weight of your body on the ground underneath you, the contact of your arms against your body. Slowly scan down your body, starting from the top of your head. Without buying into or analysing them, softly note any physical feelings or emotions that might be present, just observing them, like you would traffic passing you by. Continue down to your belly. Feel your stomach muscles relaxing as you visualize them melting away any tension with each breath. Continue scanning down your body, all the way to your toes.*

- **LET YOUR MIND REST BACK ON THE PHYSICAL SENSATION OF THE BREATH,** *noticing the rhythm and how each breath is a little different from the last. Continue for ten long, slow breaths, maintaining the curiosity as you sit with each unique breath. It is completely normal for your mind to wander off; when it does so, gently acknowledge the thought or feeling, before bringing your attention back to your breath.*

- **BRING YOUR FOCUS BACK INTO THE BODY AND YOUR SURROUNDINGS,** *noting the contact between your legs and the ground and the air on your skin. Note any background sounds or smells. Take a few breaths here. With your final deep breath, feel the oxygen filling your body, and a deeper sense of relaxation as you exhale out, this time through your nose.*

- **IN YOUR OWN TIME, AND ONLY WHEN YOU'RE READY,** *slowly open your eyes. Before you move off, take a moment to appreciate how it feels to have given yourself these fifteen minutes to reconnect with your mind, your body (and your GM, too). Shall I see you back here tomorrow?*

> *If you find this part of the flow beneficial, you might like to try one of the meditation apps such as* **Headspace** *or* **Calm**, *which offer a range of mindfulness exercises to suit different needs. Whatever you choose, the most important thing is to make this a daily habit. For those new to mindfulness, I get that, initially, the breathing and stillness can feel a little uncomfortable. However, with time, I can assure you that your mind and body will start to crave the clarity that yoga can bring.*

Exercise: Move your body

We all know exercise is good for us, but the idea that it also benefits our GM may be the extra incentive we need to get moving. While most of the current research comes from observational and animal studies, more is emerging in actual humans (go figure) suggesting that the link between exercise and a diverse GM is independent of diet. This means that it's not just because people who exercise tend to eat differently. The study also found that the benefit relied on sustained exercise, so hitting the exercise hard for a few weeks and then burning out and stopping is not going to do your GM much good in the long term.

When it comes to the type of exercise, funnily enough, your GM likes whatever you do … or perhaps they've wired us to like whatever they do. As long as you're moving your body often, getting your heart rate up for at least thirty minutes most days, you'll be satisfying everyone's needs.

Assessment : HOW ACTIVE ARE YOU?

So how do your fitness levels rate? Head to www.TheGutHealthDoctor.com to check in with how your fitness levels compare to recommendations.

Exercise is not just about training for heart fitness and perfecting our running technique, there is another side to it, a more targeted type – have you ever considered your bowel fitness or pooping technique?

This unconventional type of fitness is not to be dismissed – it has revolutionized the way in which many gut symptoms are managed, particularly constipation, urgency and incontinence (when you can't hold your poop back). What about if you don't have any symptoms? Is it still relevant? Absolutely, maintaining your bowel fitness is also helpful in the prevention of issues as we age and our pooping muscles weaken. For women who plan to conceive one day, it's even more crucial, with as many as 50 per cent of mums who give birth vaginally having issues with this.

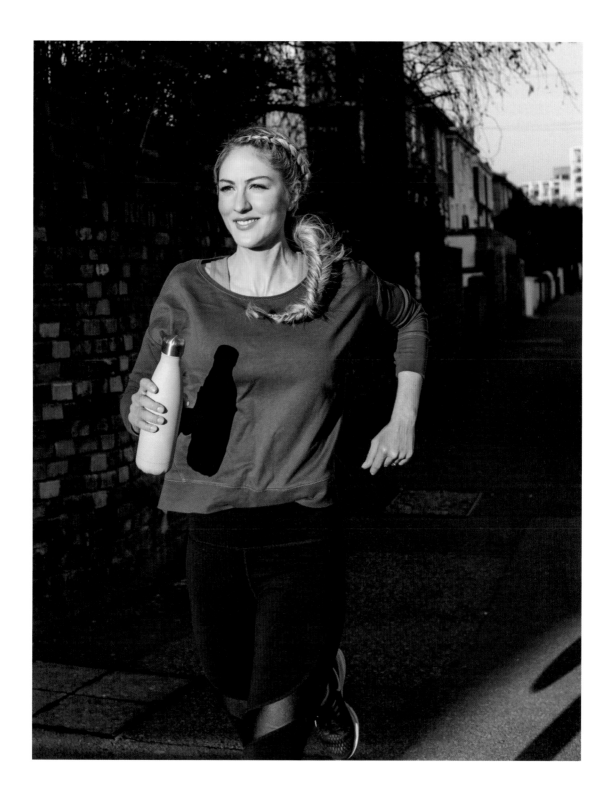

Bowel-training exercises

With the help of bowel-training expert Ellie Bradshaw and pelvic health physiotherapist Lucy Allen, we've got some basics to get your bowel fit.

Correct pooping position

Did you know that the human body was designed to poop in the squatting position? It's a fact seemingly overlooked by the masterminds behind the sitting toilet. It may also be no coincidence that countries with sitting toilets (much of the Western world) have an increased risk of pooping issues. But don't worry, guys: you don't need to let your elevated toilet define you. Here is how you can get your pooping position just right.

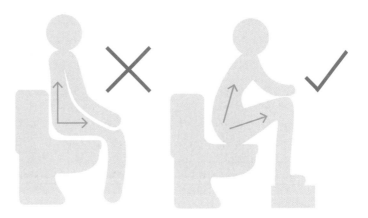

1. **WHEN SITTING ON THE TOILET, ENSURE YOUR KNEES ARE SLIGHTLY HIGHER THAN YOUR HIPS.** For this, you can utilize an old phone book or shoe box, or invest in a foot step to place under your feet.

2. **LEANING FORWARD, PROP YOUR ELBOWS ON TOP OF YOUR KNEES.**

3. **ENSURE YOUR SPINE IS STRAIGHT AND BULGE OUT YOUR TUMMY** (everything below the belly button).

4. **RELAX AND LOWER YOUR SHOULDERS.**

There you have it: the toilet position that straightens out the bottom of the intestine and the anus, the exit point, allowing for a smooth departure.

How to be a good pooper

Pooping is rather like dancing: everyone can do it, but for some of us it requires a little more effort and concentration to master the moves. How good a pooper you are is not just down to your inherent ability to coordinate the muscles but is also determined by learned behaviours from as far back as your toilet-training days.

For those struggling with constipation or incomplete evacuation (where you don't feel like you've emptied your bowels properly), follow the steps below to help ensure the appropriate coordination of your pooping muscles.

1. ONCE IN THE CORRECT POOPING POSITION, move your hands around the sides of your waist and cough. Feel your waist widen. These are the muscles to use when pooping.

2. MAKE YOURSELF AS WIDE AS POSSIBLE BY BROADENING AT THE WAIST and bulging out the lower tummy. Bear down to create the pressure and propulsion for two to three seconds, as if you are trying to force out gas. Relax a while, then repeat. Do this a few times both to initiate and complete emptying.

Many people strain from their chest, which is counterproductive. Why? This can cause tightening of your outer pooping sphincter and pelvic-floor muscles, blocking the 'exit' pathway.

If you're suffering from constipation and feel like you'd benefit from more training, chat to your GP about seeing a biofeedback specialist nurse like Ellie.

Strengthening the pelvic floor

The pelvic floor is a sheet of muscles, likened to a trampoline, extending from your tailbone to your pubic bone (back to front) and from one side of your butt bones to the other (side to side). This muscle is not only crucial for keeping our intestine (and other organs like the bladder) in place, preventing prolapses, it's also important for maintaining bowel and urine continence. Essentially, it keeps us in control of our urges and prevents any 'leaks', whether we're star-jumping in the gym or stranded without a toilet in sight.

A weak pelvic floor is very common – a third of all women experience a problem with their pelvic floor over their lifetime. Getting on top of it early will help you beat this statistic. If this is not enough of an incentive, it also improves your sex life.

How to strengthen your pelvic-floor muscles

1. TO CONTRACT YOUR PELVIC-FLOOR MUSCLES, START BY TIGHTENING YOUR BACK PASSAGE (anal sphincter), as if to stop gas coming out. Then extend the contraction, lifting up and forwards to your pubic bone, as if you are also trying to stop the flow of urine. This is your pelvic floor muscles contracted.

2. ACTIVATE AND HOLD YOUR PELVIC-FLOOR MUSCLES FOR UP TO TEN SECONDS. If you can't feel the muscle still squeezing by the ten-second mark, it means your pelvic floor is a little weak. If so, try starting with a shorter hold.

3. REPEAT STEP 1 AS MANY TIMES AS YOU CAN, relaxing for five to ten seconds in between each squeeze, until you feel the muscles starting to get tired. This may be between five and up to a maximum of fifteen repetitions.

4. NOW TRY QUICK 'SNAPS', tightening up the muscle back to front quickly, then relaxing for a few seconds, then repeating. Make sure that, in between each squeeze or snap, you fully relax the muscle, breathing naturally as you are holding. If you feel your butt clenching, your eyebrows rising or that you've forgotten to breathe, you may be trying too hard (happens to the best of us). Aim for ten to fifteen snaps each time.

If you can complete at least five of the ten-second holds, then doing these exercises once a day is enough to maintain strength and function. For those with weaker pelvic floors (less than five holds), try to do these exercises three times a day. I know it sounds like a lot, but the good thing about them is that they can essentially be done anywhere. Waiting for the train, cooking dinner, even when sitting in a meeting – no one will ever know.

> ✋ **Caution:** Not all pelvic-floor problems are fixed by strengthening them. If you have any of the problems below, it's best to get the advice of a physiotherapist, as sometimes the pelvic-floor muscles can get too tight or sensitive, causing difficulty pooping or pelvic pain.
>
> - PROLAPSE – feeling like something is coming down or out of the vagina or anus
> - DIFFICULTY EMPTYING THE BOWEL – this may also be related to poor coordination and spasming; learning to relax the pelvic floor may help
> - PELVIC PAIN – pain in your bladder or bottom pre- and post-pooping, painful sex

Bowel massage

If you think about our intestine as being coated in muscle, it makes sense that massaging the intestine, in particular the large intestine, where things can get a little sluggish and gas can become trapped, can help soothe gut symptoms. This strategy is supported by a trial which demonstrated that daily bowel massage for eight weeks was an effective addition to managing both constipation and tummy pain. The good thing about this type of massage is that it's free – you can easily do it yourself by following these simple steps, so why not give it a try? The bowel massage is best done daily and using massage oil.

> **Caution:** If you are pregnant or have a history of inflammatory bowel disease, recent scarring or abdominal surgery, spine issues or a history of colon cancer, it's best to discuss abdominal massage with your GP first.

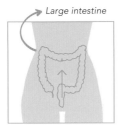
Large intestine

1. PREPARING THE GUT
Gently stroke upwards with a flat hand (3 times).

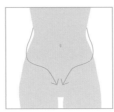

2. STIMULATING THE GUT
Stroke from your mid back firmly down the sides of your tummy into the groin (10 times).

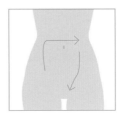

3. MOVING THINGS ALONG
Using fisted hands, stroke up and around your large intestine, with your right fist moving up, across and left fist moving down (2 minutes).

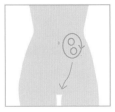

4. PUMPING DOWN
Using your fist, knead down the left side of your intestine. Imagine you're kneading dough down a tube (2 minutes).

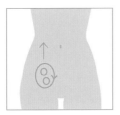

5. MOVING THINGS UP
As step 4 but moving up the right intestine (2 minutes).

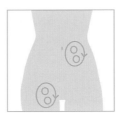

6. FINAL PUSH
Repeat steps 4 then 3.

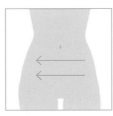

7. WINDING DOWN
Gentle stroking across with a flat hand (10 times).

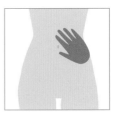

8. GAS RELEASE
Gently push down and shake with a flat hand across the large intestine (6 spots).

CHAPTER 8

In the kitchen

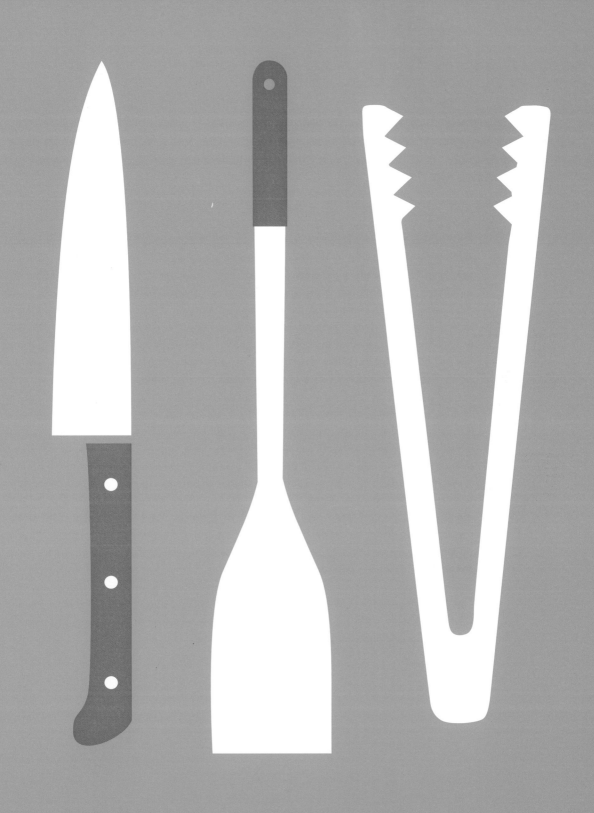

In the kitchen

Welcome to my kitchen, my favourite room in the house. This is where I see small changes making a big impact. My kitchen mission is to translate the science from lab to plate, creating delicious food that won't just make your taste buds dance but will see your gut microbes thrive too.

Food makes me very happy – I come from a big Italian family where meal times were a celebration that brought all my favourite people together. But I know it's not the same for everyone. For many of my patients, who lead busy lives or are struggling with gut issues, the thought of preparing food can provoke added stress and anxiety. If this sounds like you, I want this chapter to help change that for you. This is about reviving your passion for flavour and food; I want you to feel at ease with these recipes. They offer flexibility with intolerances, time limitations, space constraints, budgets, cooking skills – inclusivity is the name of my cooking game. I've also included my beginners' guide to fermenting and sprouting – two of my favourite activities which really do open up a whole other world of food, flavour and fun.

To start, let's revisit the concept of 'gut friendly' food. This is a rather ambiguous term because it can mean different things to different people. For example, for those without gut symptoms whose primary goal is to boost beneficial microbes, many high-FODMAP foods (which, as we discussed in Chapter 6, are high in prebiotics) are great to include. But for those with irritable bowel syndrome (IBS), large amounts may trigger symptoms. To help with this, I've added tips on how to modify the recipes, making it easy to turn any of them into a dish that fits your dietary needs according to where you are on your journey. Keep in mind that many of the restrictions we discussed in Chapters 4, 5 and 6 are only short-term tools to help identify your triggers or to give your gut a little rest while you work on settling that gut–brain axis using the strategies we looked at in Chapter 7.

The underlying theme of all the recipes is that they provide good nutrition for both you and your gut microbiota (GM), so whether the recipe is low in lactose or gluten-free, rest assured, neither your taste buds nor your GM will be missing out.

Meal planning
– building the foundation

Although not for everyone, meal planning can be a valuable tool in terms of overcoming barriers to nourishing you and your microbes. If you're struggling with this, you'll recognize that no amount of knowledge can overcome it; planning really is key. I'm certainly not talking about generic meal plans – in my ten years of experience, I've yet to meet anyone who has succeeded with one. Yes, perhaps you can stick to it for a few weeks but, as soon as life gets busy, it's usually the first thing to go. My no-generic-meal-plan approach is not always popular when I first suggest it to patients who walk in with their heart set on one. However, they quickly discover that a generic plan simply doesn't work, and it's because only you know the ins and outs of your life within which eating is entwined. You're the only one who can create a plan that can withstand the challenges of your unique life.

BUT DON'T WORRY, YOU'RE NOT ON YOUR OWN: this chapter offers guidance and inspiration to help get you started. On the next page is the template my patients who are struggling with this barrier use to create their own tailored plans. You'll see that I've also included a space to record your planning and shopping day. I know this may sound a little regimented but, for many, having this structure for around nine weeks (remember: it's thought that's the average time to form a habit, according to research from University College London) can turn meal planning from feeling like a taxing obligation into second nature. Looking after your GM is a marathon, not a sprint – we're looking for long-term changes. However, if you prefer to start off with a sprint, to build your motivation and momentum, by all means sprint away – just keep a gauge on your fuel tank along the way.

I have filled out Monday as an example of what one day might look like.

	Breakfast	Lunch	Dinner	Snacks*	Drinks
Monday	DIY granola (page 201)	Mix-and-match slider (page 210)	Meatless meatballs in rich tomato sauce (page 234)	Sea salt and rosemary legume crunch (page 246)	Water (1.5l) 1 shot of coffee Water kefir (page 276)
Tuesday					
Wednesday					
Thursday					
Friday					
Saturday					
Sunday					
Plant-based diversity**					
Planning day			**Shopping day**		

Remember to be realistic: include some of your faves.

** *Did you reach your thirty different plant-based foods? Remember, from Chapter 3, that our GM craves plant diversity.*

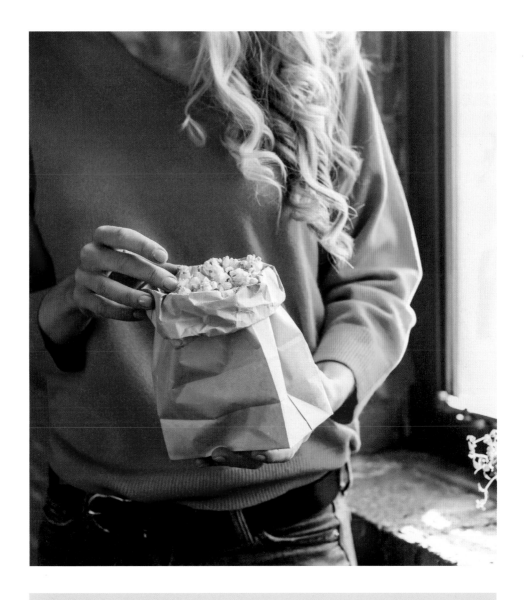

Snacks on the run

- Naked fruit

- Naked nuts and seeds

- Live natural yoghurt

- Popcorn au naturel

- As a general guide, products with at least 3g fibre/100g, no added sugar on the ingredients list and salt content of 0.3g/100g or less (or sodium 0.1g/100g or less)

Recipe modifications

Modification	Ingredient	Replacement
GLUTEN-FREE	Soy sauce	• Tamari (double-check on the label that it doesn't contain wheat) • Gluten-free soy sauce
	Baking powder	• Gluten-free baking powder
	Grains/pasta	See page 127
	Spelt, wholegrain wheat flour	• Wholegrain gluten-free flour • Combine 50 per cent brown rice flour, 25 per cent cornflour, 25 per cent almond meal
FODMAP-lite* * See page 152 for the FODMAP-lite approach. For those following the full FODMAP approach, see your dietitian for a comprehensive list of high- and low-FODMAP foods.	Garlic, onion	• Pickled • Garlic-infused oil (strained) • Asafoetida powder (best 'fried off' in the pan with a touch of oil before adding other ingredients) • Green part of spring onion • Chives
	Additional herbs and spices	• Allspice, basil, capers, cinnamon, coriander, cumin, curry powder, dill, ginger, lemon, lime, mint, mustard, nutmeg, paprika, parsley, pepper, rosemary, thyme, turmeric and vanilla
LOW-LACTOSE		See page 129
DAIRY-FREE	Yoghurt	Plant-based yoghurt (coconut, soya, etc.)
	Cow's milk	Plant-based milks* (soya, rice, oat, almond)

*Opt for calcium-fortified. Cow's milk cannot be substituted for plant-based milks in the fermenting recipes.

Modification	Ingredient	Replacement
OTHER	Self-raising flour	120g plain flour + 1 tsp baking powder
	Egg	• (for binding) **Flax-egg:** 1 tbsp ground flaxseed with 3 tbsp warm water; stir and let set for 15 minutes • (for binding) **Chia-egg:** 1 tbsp chia seeds with 3 tbsp warm water; stir and let set for 15 minutes • (for thickening) **Arrowroot:** 1 tbsp • (most purposes) **Egg-replacer:** (made from blended flours, raising agents and gums), available from most health-food shops
	Nuts	• **Toppings:** legume crunch (page 246), crumbled seeded crackers (page 245), dried fruit • **Butters:** sunflower seed, pumpkin seed • **Coatings:** polenta, rolled oats, breadcrumbs • **Added texture:** finely diced celery, beansprouts, chopped spring onion
	Cheese	• Cashew cheese (page 213) • Plant-based cheeses (soya, almond, etc.) • Nutritional yeast (see box below)

◆ *What's the deal with nutritional yeast? Although similar to the yeast used to make bread and brew beer, the function of nutritional yeast is very different. The yeast is not alive, so it doesn't do any fermenting. Instead, it is used to add flavour (a delicious cheesy, nutty taste) and nutrition. Nutritional yeast is an excellent source of B vitamins (including B12 when fortified) and is rich in fibre and protein. Because of this, fortified nutritional yeast is considered a dietary staple for those whose diet is 100 per cent plant-based.*

Breakfast

For me, there really is something special about breakfast. Whether it's creamy kefir oats, some granola crunch, light and fluffy pancakes, perfectly gooey eggs or a warm breakfast loaf, it's all part of my breakfast love affair. For those who need a bit more convincing, breakfast not only physically sets your gut up for the day, triggering that gastrocolic reflex (which gets 'things' moving), if you're feeding your GM (think fibre, plant diversity), breakfast has been shown to increase mental and physical alertness, too. Psychologically, kicking your day off with a nutritious start can lay down a strong, positive foundation for the rest of the day. For those who are still a little unsure, keep in mind that there are no breakfast rules – it doesn't need to be big if you're not hungry, or eaten as soon as you wake up if you're into the longer fasts. You can also prevent it becoming a time-consuming full-on event if your mornings are a little chaotic, with my breakfast on the run options. Do breakfast your way, just try not to miss out on what it has to offer.

My breakfast staple (fermented overnight oats)

There is something comforting about going to bed knowing that millions of microbes will continue working through the night, transforming your breakfast into a flavour-infused jar of goodness. This recipe doesn't just offer live microbes, but a sizeable 8 grams of fibre per portion.

Base:
45g rolled oats
1 tsp mixed seeds
1 tbsp chia seeds
1 tbsp desiccated coconut
1 extra-ripe banana, mashed (100g peeled weight)
50ml dairy kefir (see page 274)
200ml soy milk, or milk of choice
1 Medjool date, thinly chopped, or sweetener of choice

Toppers (choose 1 to add to your base):

CARROT CAKE:
½ a small carrot, grated (40g prepped weight)
1 tbsp walnuts, crushed
½ tsp cinnamon

COCOA AND COURGETTE:
¼ a small courgette, grated (40g prepped weight)
2 tsp cocoa powder
1 tbsp dark-chocolate shavings

1. In a mixing bowl, combine all base and topper ingredients of choice and stir well.

2. Divide into two 300ml jars and cover with the lid.

3. Leave in a warm (around 25°C, or on a heat mat), dark place overnight to allow the kefir microbes to work their magic, infusing the flavours throughout.

4. After 8 hours, stir through. Breakfast is served. Pop the second jar in the fridge for tomorrow's breakfast.

Options:
• Not ready for fermenting? Replace the kefir with your milk of choice and leave in the fridge overnight.

◆ *As the microbes from the kefir prepare your breakfast, that is, ferment it, they produce beneficial organic acids, which are a little tart-tasting. I crave that tart bite, but if you're new to fermenting you may want to shorten the fermenting time and build up. This recipe also works best using home-made kefir from grains (see page 274).*

Breakfast on the run

Serves 1

Don't let those manic mornings get in the way of a tasty and nutritious breakfast for you and your GM. These are some of my fast favourites and have saved me from many sugar-overloaded breakfast bars and shop-bought buttery pastries that never quite seem to hit the mark.

MONDAY

Two-minute scram

2 large eggs, whisked
2 tbsp milk
1 tbsp fresh herbs, finely chopped (or spring onions)
1 slice grainy bread, roughly chopped
6 cherry tomatoes, halved

1. Swirl one large mug (or bowl) with a touch of oil, then add all the ingredients. Season to taste and, as an option, shake in mixed seeds. Roughly mix.

Note: The egg will rise when cooking so ensure the mug/bowl is no more than half full.

2. Cook on high in the microwave for 1 minute. Stir. Return for a further minute or until the egg has set.

TUESDAY

Live breakfast parfait

200g live thick yoghurt (page 280)
50g berries of choice
40g granola mix (page 201)
1 tbsp dark chocolate, shaved

1. Layer a serving glass with the top 3 ingredients: spoon in half the yoghurt, then half the fruit, then half the cereal, and repeat.

2. Top with chocolate shavings.

WEDNESDAY

Thick protein shake

110g silken tofu
1 large banana, frozen
250ml dairy kefir (see page 274)
1 tsp cinnamon

1. Put all the ingredients into a blender and buzzzzz until smooth. (You may need to add some milk of choice if it's too thick; alternatively, just eat it like ice cream!)

Optional: shake seeds or a spoon of granola mix (page 201) on top.

THURSDAY

Avocado and feta slider

½ a tomato, thinly sliced
¼ an avocado, thinly sliced
2 wholegrain crackers (page 245)
30g feta cheese
a shake of mixed seeds

1. Lay the tomato slices then the avocado across the crackers before crumbling the feta on top, sprinkling with seeds and seasoning to taste.

Peanut and pear open sandwich

1 pear, cut along its
 length into 6–7 slices
2 tbsp peanut butter
2 tbsp live thick
 yoghurt (page 280)
a shake of mixed
 seeds

1. Spread the peanut
butter across a slice
of pear, add some
yoghurt and top
with seeds. Eat and
repeat.

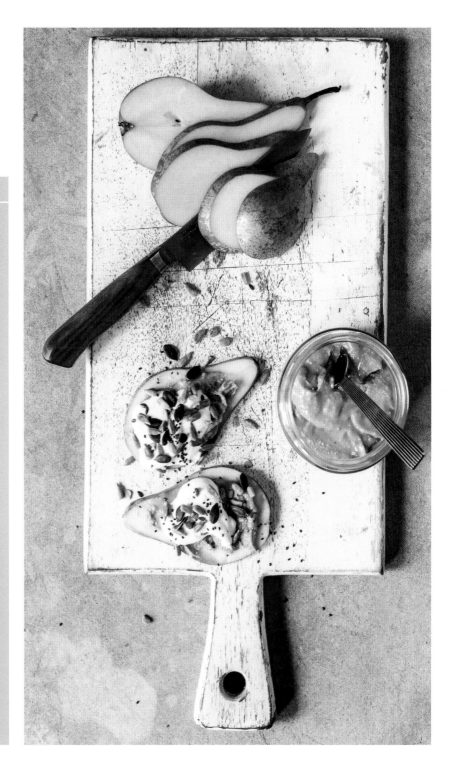

Mix-and-match porridge

Many of us tend to eat the same breakfast on repeat, making it a rather boring meal. This DIY breakfast template is all about inspiring you to mix things up and get creative. Build the ultimate breakfast by choosing one ingredient per box. Stir together, and enjoy! The portions are just there as a guide, but remember it's your breakfast! Adjust according to your taste preferences.

Fibre base

(40g) – the base way to kick things off
Raw grains typically double in size when cooked; if starting with raw, use 40g. If choosing cooked options, for ultimate convenience, buy precooked grains, which require no more than 1–2 minutes in the microwave (cooked grain approx. 80g); otherwise, cook according to packet instructions.

- Rolled oats
- Wheat flakes
- Buckwheat (cooked)
- Amaranth (cooked)
- Quinoa (cooked)

Polyphenol hit

(50g) – those GM-loving plant chemicals

- Strawberries, sliced
- Blueberries
- Apple, grated
- Pear, sliced
- Chickpeas
- Cherry tomatoes

Hydration

(100–150ml) – after all, our body is over 50 per cent water by weight

- Cow's milk
- Soya milk*
- Oat milk*
- Almond milk*
- Side of tea

Consider opting for calcium-fortified varieties.

Flavour punch

rewarding your taste buds for getting you out of bed

- Coconut flakes (1 tbsp) & vanilla extract (¼ tsp)
- Cinnamon (½ tsp) & nutmeg (pinch)
- Grated ginger & cinnamon (½ tsp each)
- Dark-chocolate chips (1 tbsp)
- Feta cheese (1 tbsp)

Live culture

(2 tbsp) – some more microbes to add to your mix

- Live thick yoghurt (page 280)
- Dairy kefir (page 274)
- Live coconut yoghurt
- Coconut kefir
- Kimchi (page 270)

Prebiotic boost

(1 tbsp) – a real treat for the best-behaved microbes

- Dried figs, thinly sliced
- Dates or prunes, thinly sliced
- Dried apricots, diced
- Cashews
- Pomegranate

Healthy fats

(1 tbsp) – fuelling a healthy heart and mind

- Walnuts
- Almond butter
- Pistachios
- Chia seeds
- Avocado

Power plant pancakes

Breakfast is often a missed opportunity when it comes to contributing to your five portions of vegetables per day – something these pancakes will put a stop to. But they don't just deliver on veg, they're also a real treat for the taste buds.

Base:
150g sweet potato, roughly chopped
60g rolled oats
75g tinned cannellini beans, drained and rinsed
1 large extra-ripe banana (120g peeled weight)
250ml soy milk, or milk of choice
4 large eggs, whisked
1 tsp cinnamon
1 tsp vanilla extract
1 tsp baking powder
Olive oil, or oil of choice, for frying

Toppers:
BERRY SAUCE:
160g strawberries, diced
1 medjool date, sliced

120g thick live natural yoghurt (see page 280)
1 tbsp mixed seeds

1. Place the sweet potato and a small splash of water into a microwave-safe dish. Cover and cook on high for 4 minutes.

2. Prepare the berry sauce. In a small saucepan, combine the strawberries, the date and 125ml of water and bring to a gentle boil. Using the back of a spatula, squish the strawberries and chopped dates, then simmer for 10 minutes.

3. Meanwhile, once the sweet potato has cooled, blend together with all the base ingredients, except the oil, to form a smooth batter.

4. In a non-stick frying pan, warm a little oil over a low-medium heat. Add a quarter of a cup (60ml) of the batter to it. Cook for 3 minutes or so until there are bubbles in the pancake and you can lift it to flip easily.

5. Flip and cook on the other side for 1–2 minutes. Remove from the pan to a plate and cover with a clean cloth to keep warm.

6. Repeat the process with the rest of the batter. Serve the pancakes, drizzled with berry sauce, a dollop of yoghurt and a sprinkling of seeds.

◆ *Oats are a great source of beta-glucans, a type of fibre. There is strong evidence for their health benefits which include lowering cholesterol and managing sugar levels in people with diabetes. They've also been shown to help regulate our appetite, making us less likely to grab for the biscuit barrel.*

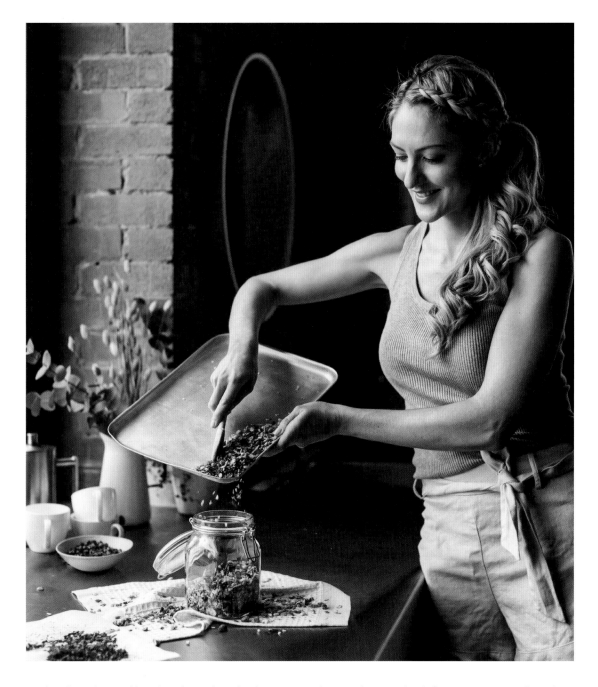

◆ *The phytochemical betalain that is found in beetroot is what you have to thank for turning your milk pink. Better still, betalain has been shown to be a powerful antioxidant with anti-cancer properties, at least in animal studies.*

DIY granola

After searching high and low, I still couldn't find a granola that ticked the boxes for both flavour and nutrition. So I decided to make my own gut-loving mix, and I haven't looked back! I make a batch every fortnight on a Sunday and use it as both a breakfast and as a snack, adding that all-important crunch to my yoghurt. You'll also be getting close to a third of your daily fibre needs from each portion.

Base:
110g jumbo oats (or muesli mix of choice)
20g coconut flakes
70g mixed seeds (linseed, sunflower, pumpkin, sesame)
70g almonds, chopped
½ tbsp olive oil
½ tsp cinnamon
½ tsp nutmeg
½ tsp vanilla extract
2 Medjool dates, stirred into a paste with 1 tbsp boiling water, or sweetener of choice
2 tsp ground ginger (optional)

Toppers (optional):
400g tinned lentils, drained and rinsed
1 raw beetroot, grated
25g goji berries
45g dried figs, sliced
55g dried apricots, sliced

1. Preheat the oven to 150°C fan/325°F/gas mark 3.

2. In a large bowl, combine the oats, coconut flakes, seeds and almonds.

3. In a small bowl, mix together the olive oil, cinnamon, nutmeg, vanilla extract and date paste, and the ginger, if using, before pouring over the dry ingredients. Using your hands, mix together to coat evenly. Set aside.

4. Thinly spread the mix across two baking trays lined with baking paper. Pop in the oven for 10 minutes, toss, then continue baking for a further 10 minutes, or until golden. If you are including the lentils or beetroot, pat dry before laying on separate trays and place in the oven alongside the granola mix (20 minutes for the beetroot, 30 minutes for the lentils, or until dry and crisp).

5. Remove from the oven and sprinkle on your toppers of choice. Allow to cool before placing in an airtight container. Serve with some live yoghurt and milk of your choice.

Options:
• Like a chunkier granola? Add 30ml of water and double the oil and dates, press into the tray and bake for an extra 5–10 minutes.
• Experiment with different grains, nuts and dried fruit to introduce more diversity into your diet.

Chickpea crêpes with creamy feta and fungi

Proof that a glamorous dish full of flavour doesn't need to cost you your whole morning in prep or cleaning – it really is the perfect way to start your weekend.

Base:

50g gram flour (also known as chickpea or besan flour)
½ tsp garlic powder
pinch of salt
a twist of pepper
15g pickled beetroot or spinach leaves
olive oil, or oil of choice, for frying

Toppers:

1 tbsp olive oil
200g mushrooms, chopped
1 clove of garlic, thinly sliced
¼ tsp rosemary or thyme (optional)
60g live thick yoghurt or hummus (see pages 280 & 240)
40g feta, crumbled
150g cherry tomatoes, halved
a sprinkle of seeds
a poached egg or a slice of smoked salmon (optional)

The crêpe:

1. In a blender, put the flour, spices, seasoning, 120ml of water and the beetroot or spinach. Blitz for 30 seconds. Set the thin batter aside for 30 minutes in a warm place to allow the flour to hydrate while you prep the toppers and do your morning yoga flow (see page 171).

2. Warm a little oil over a medium heat in a non-stick frying pan. Add one third of a cup (75ml) of the batter to the pan.

3. Cook for approximately 2–3 minutes, until there are bubbles in the crêpe and you can lift it over to flip easily.

4. Flip and cook on the other side for 1–2 minutes.

5. Remove from the pan to a plate and cover with a clean cloth to keep warm. Repeat the process with the remaining batter.

The toppers:

6. Heat the oil in the frying pan then add the mushrooms and garlic. Stir together and sauté for 2–3 minutes until soft and slightly browned. Add any optional fresh herbs and season to taste.

7. Line your crêpe with a dollop of yoghurt or hummus, a layer of warm mushrooms and a crumble of feta. Top with cherry tomatoes, seeds and egg or salmon, if desired, before folding the crêpe and tucking in.

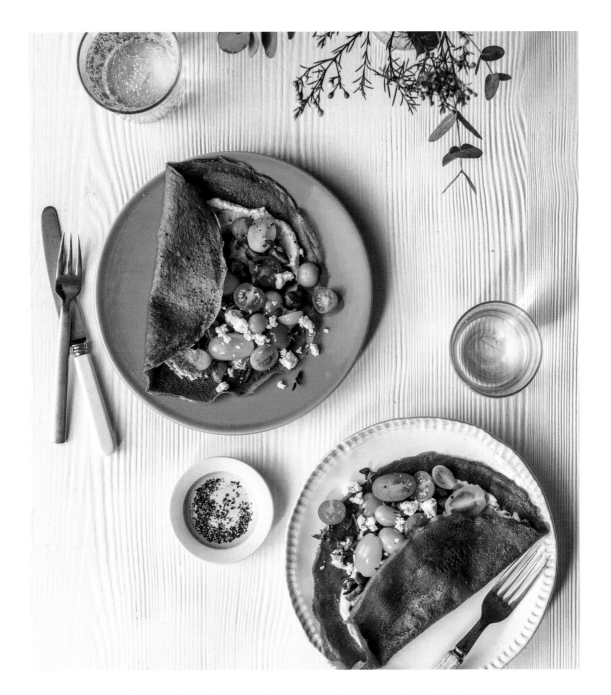

◆ *Similarly to the way in which our skin can make vitamin D when exposed to sunlight (UV light), so too can mushrooms. In winter I keep my mushrooms on my kitchen window sill, exposed to sunlight, to maximize my vitamin D intake. Vitamin D is crucial not only for strong bones but for our mental health too.*

Serves 4

Mini shakshuka egg pots

After making these beauties, you'll never be tempted to order baked eggs out again.

Base:
3 peppers, mixed colours
1 tbsp olive oil
6 spring onions, chopped
4 cloves of garlic, thinly
    sliced
1 tsp cumin seeds
200g tinned butter-
    beans, drained and
    rinsed
6 tomatoes, chopped
chilli flakes
a handful of coriander,
    chopped
2 tbsp black olives,
    chopped (optional)
2 tbsp capers (optional)
4 mini wholegrain wraps
    (see page 247)
salt and pepper

Toppers:
4 large eggs
3 tbsp live thick yoghurt
    (see page 280)
seeded crackers (optional,
    see pages 243–5)

1. Preheat the oven to 170°C fan/375°F/gas mark 5.

2. In a griddle pan, chargrill the peppers over a high heat for approximately 15 minutes, turning frequently until nice and charred on both sides. Set aside and, when cooled, chop into small pieces.

3. In a non-stick frying pan, warm the oil over a medium heat. Add the spring onions, garlic and cumin. Fry until soft and slightly browned. Add the butterbeans, tomatoes, peppers, chilli flakes and coriander, and the olives and capers, if using, and season to taste. Simmer for 10–15 minutes, or until soft. Note: you may need to add a little water if the mixture gets too dry.

4. Line each of four ramekins (or ovenproof mugs) with a mini wrap to act as the shakshuka case.

5. Divide the shakshuka between each ramekin, making a well in the middle before cracking an egg into each one.

6. Place the ramekins on a baking tray and bake for 8–10 minutes, or until the whites are set but the yolks are still runny. Top with a dollop of yoghurt and enjoy warm with crackers to dip in.

◆ *Ever wondered why some egg yolks are darker than others? The delicious deep-orange colour is all thanks to the higher levels of the phytochemical beta-carotene. Studies have found that free-range chickens often produce eggs with higher levels of beta-carotene, as well as other nutrients such as omega-3. Why? Free-range chickens graze not only on grass, seeds and weeds but also on worms and insects, which makes their diet more nutrient dense.*

Spicy baked beans

I didn't think I was that into baked beans until my friend Niki (who I call the flavour queen) opened my eyes to these flavours. Now I always make a double batch and add them into my gut-goodness bowls (see page 222) the next day. I also freeze into single portions and reheat as a snack. In terms of prebiotic load, this dish is hard to beat, and sports 10 grams of total fibre per portion.

Base:
2 tbsp olive oil
1 onion, diced
3 cloves of garlic, crushed
1 tsp smoked paprika
½ tsp cayenne pepper
1 tsp cumin seeds
1 x 400g tin of tomatoes
4 sundried tomatoes, preserved in oil
1 x 400g tin of borlotti beans, drained and rinsed
1 x 400g tin of cannellini beans, drained and rinsed
40g black olives, sliced (optional)
1 tbsp tamari or soy sauce
1 tsp sweetener of choice
1 tsp vinegar of choice
40g spinach leaves, washed (optional)
1 tsp chilli flakes (optional)
salt and pepper

Toppers (optional):
8 eggs, poached/fried/scrambled
live thick yoghurt or hummus (see pages 280 & 240)
small handful of alfalfa sprouts

1. In a non-stick frying pan, warm the oil over a low–medium heat. Add the onion, garlic and spices and sauté for a few minutes.

2. Add the tinned tomatoes and sundried tomatoes and simmer for 15 minutes on a low heat.

3. Add in the beans, and olives, if using, and cook for a further 15 minutes.

4. Finally, add the tamari or soy sauce, sweetener, vinegar, and the spinach leaves and chilli, if using. Simmer for a few minutes. Season to taste.

5. Plate the beans and top with eggs and a dollop of yoghurt, hummus or both. Sprinkle on the alfalfa sprouts, if using.

◆ *Considering skipping the oil? A trial compared the impact of eating cooked tomatoes with and without olive oil for five days. Those who included the oil had significantly greater levels of the phytochemical lycopene in their blood. Tomatoes + heat + olive oil = higher lycopene bioavailability. Why do we care about lycopene? Not only has it been shown to increase your skin's defence against the sun (although that's still not an excuse to skip sunscreen), it is linked with better heart health and a lower risk of prostate cancer.*

Banana, fig and courgette breakfast loaf

This is one of my favourite 'accidental' creations. Throwing in a bit of this and a bit of that turned into something pretty magical. The loaf was devoured within an hour (I promise, I did share) and, thanks to all your requests on social media, I decided to repeat the 'accident' the next day, this time measuring out all the ingredients so that I could share it with you. Offering over 5 grams of fibre per portion, you'll be hard pressed to find a loaf to match.

Base:
100g teff grain
120g wholewheat spelt flour
2 tsp baking powder
2 tsp cinnamon
a pinch of salt
40ml olive oil
3 large eggs
2 tsp vanilla extract
3 extra-ripe bananas, mashed (300g peeled weight)
70g dried figs, diced
½ a small courgette, grated (80g prepped weight)
1 large carrot, grated (100g prepped weight)
50g walnuts, roughly chopped

Toppers:
1 banana (100g peeled weight)
10g coconut flakes (optional)

1. Preheat the oven to 170°C fan/375°F/gas mark 5.

2. In a large mixing bowl, combine all the dry ingredients (teff, spelt, baking powder, cinnamon and salt).

3. In a separate bowl, whisk together the wet ingredients (olive oil, eggs and vanilla extract) with an electric beater before adding the fruit, vegetables and nuts (bananas, figs, courgette, carrot, walnuts). Fold in the dry mixture.

4. Line a loaf tin (approx. 23 x 13cm) with baking paper, then pour in the cake mixture. Top with banana halves any way you fancy and coconut flakes, if using.

5. Pop in the oven for 70 minutes, or until cooked through. Cover with foil after 30 minutes of cooking to prevent burning the coconut. Allow to cool for 5 minutes in the tin, before lifting out with the baking paper on to a wire rack to cool completely before cutting.

◆ *Teff grain is a traditional staple in Ethiopia. This tiny gluten-free grain packs quite a nutritional punch, offering 10 grams of protein and 7 grams of fibre per cooked cup. It also offers a slightly sweet taste with undertones of cocoa and hazelnut. You can buy it from most health food stores or readily online.*

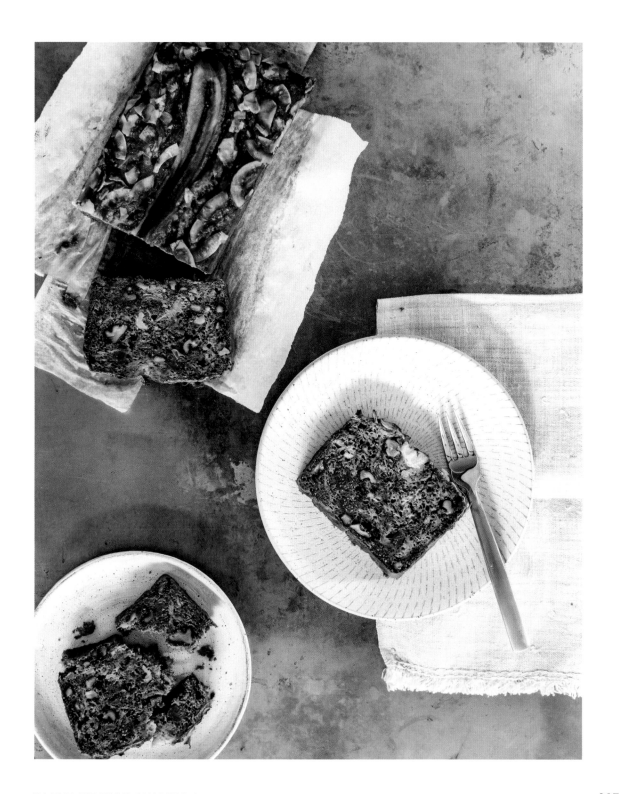

Lunch

Even if you don't live in a siesta-loving part of the world, lunch doesn't need to be a boring cut sandwich, a tasteless bag of leaves or an expensive impulse buy. Here I share five-minute 'mix-and-match' slider ideas, convenient double-batch lunch-box recipes and my GM-loving version of sushi that'll have you (and your colleagues) wishing you'd packed extras. For those times when you're looking for a more leisurely lunch which will have your guests raving about it for weeks, you may be tempted by the Korean BBQ squash tacos or the raw lasagne, which are both bursting with flavours that I'm yet to match with their meat rivals.

Sweet potato and pulsing frittata

Serves 6

When I was developing this recipe I set myself two criteria: to max out on plant-based diversity and to make it so tasty that even kids come back for seconds. Boasting twenty-one different plant-based ingredients and the 'more' approval from my two-year-old nephew – mission accomplished.

Base:
65g banana flour
65g wholemeal spelt flour
55g jumbo oats
1 tsp baking powder
1 tsp smoked paprika
a pinch of salt
6 large eggs
70ml olive oil
2 courgettes, grated
   (340g prepped weight)
½ a large sweet potato,
   grated (130g prepped
   weight)
1 onion, diced
150g mixed pre-sliced
   stir-fry vegetables
   (e.g. cabbage, carrot,
   mushroom, sprouts)
65g tinned lentils, rinsed
   and drained
80g tinned chickpeas,
   rinsed and drained
40g capers
fresh parsley, chopped
   (optional)

Toppers (optional):
1 tomato
50g feta, crumbled
2 tbsp mixed seeds
1 tsp chilli flakes

1. Preheat the oven to 170°C fan/375°F/gas mark 5.

2. In a large mixing bowl, combine all the dry ingredients (banana flour, spelt, oats, baking powder, paprika and salt).

3. In a separate bowl, whisk together the eggs and the olive oil with electric beaters until light and fluffy on top. Add in the vegetables (courgettes, sweet potato, onion, mixed vegetables, lentils, chickpeas, capers and the feta). Fold in the dry mixture.

4. Grease a flan tin (approx. 30cm diameter), then pour in the mixture. If using, top with sliced tomato; dot with feta and sprinkle with mixed seeds and chilli flakes.

5. Pop in the oven for 45–50 minutes, or until cooked through. Allow to cool for 5 minutes in the tin, before turning out on to a wire rack to cool completely.

Options:
• Banana flour is a great source of gut-loving resistant starch and is oh so tasty, but if you don't have any, replace with 90g of plain flour.

◆ *Imperfection is in, perfection is out. Plants produce phytochemicals in response to stress. This is thought to be why some 'ugly' fruit and vegetables, which have been subject to more stress, contain more phytochemicals. This is a great recipe to use up any stressed or bruised vegetables.*

Mix-and-match sliders

Select one ingredient per box. Use the portions as just a guide – it's your lunch, after all.

1. Cook the items as described or according to packet instructions. Grill foods with a drizzle of olive oil.

2. Assemble the ingredients according to your chosen wholegrain 'plate':
   a. **Wraps:** Starting with any spreads, place all the ingredients on the wrap, roll, slice and serve.
   b. **Crackers:** Build an open sandwich and make a side salad with the leftovers.

Wholegrain plate
- Wrap
- Seedy oat cakes (page 243)
- Cheesy vegan crackers (page 245)
- Spiced chickpea and sesame seed crackers (page 245)
- Fermented wrap (page 273)

Fibre base
(1 cup total)
- Courgette (grilled) Butternut squash (sliced thin, grilled)
- Mixed leaves Tomato (sliced)
- Alfalfa sprouts (page 278) Radishes (sliced)
- Pepper (grilled) Rocket leaves
- Bean shoots Swiss chard (steamed)

Prebiotic boost
(to taste)
- Pomegranate seeds
- Beetroot (grated)
- Fennel bulb (sliced)
- Asparagus (grilled)
- Savoy cabbage (shredded)

Protein punch
(50–70g)
- Hummus (page 240)
- Tofu of choice (firm, silken, smoked) (grilled)
- Eggs (boiled)
- White meat of choice (chicken, turkey, pork) (grilled)
- Legume of choice (e.g. split or green lentils)

Live kick
(1–2 tbsp)
- Live thick yoghurt (page 280)
- Aged cheese
- Raw-slaw (page 268)
- Olives
- Kimchi (page 270)

Healthy fats
(1 tbsp)
- Pine nuts
- Avocado
- Cashew cheese (page 213)
- Sprinkle of mixed seeds
- Walnuts

Flavour kick
(stir together)
- Smoky paprika (1/8 tsp) Extra virgin olive oil (1/2 tbsp)
- Cider vinegar (1/2 tsp) Balsamic vinegar (1/2 tsp) Extra virgin olive oil (1/2 tbsp) Cracked pepper
- Lemon juice (1 tbsp) Extra virgin olive oil (1/2 tbsp) Cracked pepper
- Pesto (page 214) (1 tbsp)
- Natural yoghurt (60g) Wholegrain mustard seeds (2 tsp)

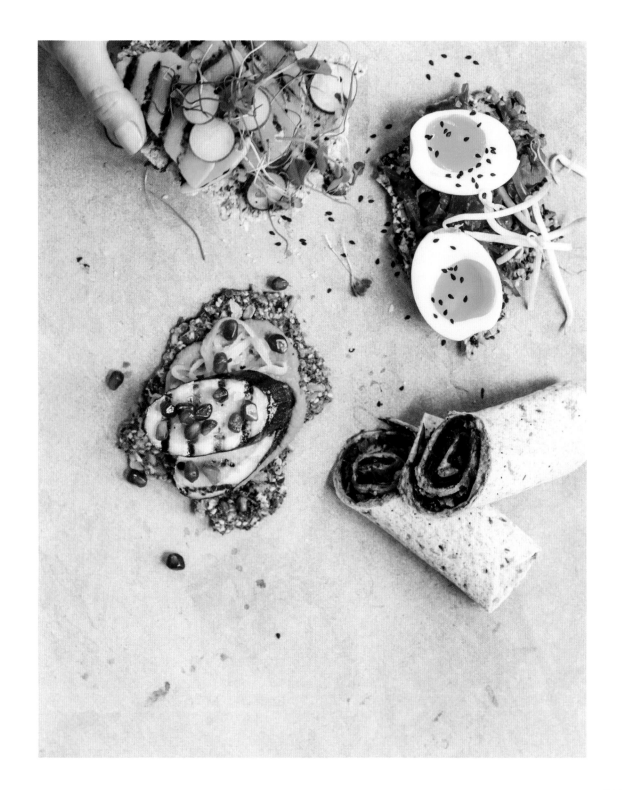

Pearl couscous in chicory boats

Inspired by my love of pintxo (tapas) and Mediterranean flavours, this is my go-to dish when I have friends over for lunch. It's loaded with fructans, a type of GM-loving prebiotic, and I've been asked for the recipe so many times that I finally decided to write it down.

Base:

1 tsp olive oil

75g pearl/Israeli couscous or grain of choice

200g cherry tomatoes, halved

¼ a red onion, sliced

200g tinned chickpeas, drained and rinsed

50g pomegranate seeds

50g artichoke, chargrilled and chopped

25g walnuts, chopped

35g Kalamata olives, pitted

9 baby mozzarella balls or 60g feta, crumbled

100g smoked fish of choice (optional)

1 large chicory head or gem lettuce, divided into leaves

Toppers:

110g live thick yoghurt (see page 280)

¼ a cucumber, grated or diced

1 tsp olive oil

1 clove of garlic, crushed

1 tbsp mint, fresh and finely sliced

a pinch of salt

1. Put the olive oil into a small saucepan over a medium heat, add the couscous and sauté for 3 minutes, or until golden brown. Add 300ml of boiling water and a pinch of salt and cook according to packet instructions (typically, 8–10 minutes). When al dente, drain and set aside to cool. Place in the fridge to cool completely.

2. Place the remaining base ingredients, apart from the chicory, into a large bowl, combine, then add the cooled couscous. Season to taste.

3. Combine the topper ingredients to make your tzatziki dressing. Taste and adjust the seasoning, if necessary.

4. Layer each chicory 'boat' with a dollop of tzatziki dressing, then scoop in the couscous mix.

Options:

• Looking to expand your grain diversity? Replace half the couscous with barley.
• Craving some more creaminess? Layer some hummus on top of the tzatziki.

◆ *Couscous cooked al dente, which means 'to the tooth', or to be firm to bite, not only tastes better but contains resistant starch, a type of fibre that your GM love. This recipe further boosts the resistant starch in the dish because the couscous is served cold. Just like potato, cooking and cooling couscous increases its resistant starch.*

Raw lasagne

Serves 4

I often get asked whether it's best to eat vegetables raw or cooked. As you guys have probably realized by now, nutrition is never black and white. Take tomatoes, for example. Cooking can destroy some nutrients (such as vitamin C) but it increases the availability of other beneficial phytochemicals (such as lycopene, linked with skin health). The best thing is to mix it up: sometimes go raw, sometimes go cooked. Here's a tasty raw lasagne to get you started.

Base:
2 large courgettes
4 tomatoes, thinly sliced

Toppers:
CASHEW CHEESE:
140g cashews
10g nutritional yeast
1 tbsp lemon juice, fresh
2 cloves of garlic
½ tbsp Dijon mustard
a pinch of salt

SPINACH AND WALNUT PESTO:
40g raw spinach leaves
40g whole basil leaves
50g walnuts
2 tsp lemon juice, fresh
1 clove of garlic
5g nutritional yeast
2 tbsp extra virgin olive oil
a pinch of salt, or to taste

1. Place all the cashew-cheese ingredients into a blender along with 120ml of warm water. Blend for 2–3 minutes until smooth. Taste and adjust salt as needed. Set aside.

2. Rinse the blender with water, then add all the pesto ingredients. Blitz until everything is combined to your preferred texture. You may need to scrape any mixture that has risen up the sides a few times. Add a dash more oil, if needed.

3. Using a mandolin or potato peeler, slice the courgettes into strips. On each serving plate, place a few slices of courgette, followed by the cheese, the tomato slices and, finally, the pesto. Repeat the layering, starting with the courgette. Aim for 2–3 layers, finishing with the cashew cheese on top. Garnish with extra basil leaves, cherry tomatoes and cracked pepper to serve.

Options:
Have your own favourite lasagne recipe? Why not switch some of the dairy cheese for this plant-based cashew version?

◆ *Leafy greens, including spinach and basil, are a great source of the phytochemicals lutein and zeaxanthin. Not only are these widely recognized as important for eye health, but in a trial they've also been shown to improve how quickly our brains process what we're seeing. This suggests they might help prevent the decline in our brain function as we age.*

Sautéed Brussels sprouts and tenderstem broccoli with pesto and wild rice

Whoever thinks 'greens' means boring needs to try this. Full of prebiotics, this cruciferous duo is good enough to convert any anti-greens advocate and will also have their GM singing out for seconds, boasting close to 8 grams of fibre per portion.

Topper (pesto):
40g basil, fresh
2 tbsp pine nuts (20g)
2 tbsp walnuts (20g)
60ml extra virgin olive oil
3 tsp Parmesan (approx. 10g), grated
1 clove of garlic
a pinch of salt, more to taste

Base:
400g wild rice, or grain/s of choice, cooked (approx. 140g raw, or use pre-cooked grain)
1 tbsp extra virgin olive oil
2 cloves of garlic, chopped
280g firm tofu, or protein of choice, cut into strips
125g Brussels sprouts, halved
200g tenderstem broccoli, quartered
250g mushrooms, halved

1. Place all the pesto ingredients into a food processor and blitz roughly until combined to your preferred texture. You may need to scrape down any mixture that has risen up the sides a few times.

2. Cook the rice according to packet instructions.

3. Meanwhile, place a frying pan over a medium heat and add the oil and garlic from the base ingredients. Fry for 1–2 minutes, then add in the tofu (or protein of choice). Fry on both sides for 5 minutes, or until light brown.

4. Remove from the frying pan, then, in the same pan, place the Brussels sprouts, broccoli, mushrooms, and a dash of water (approx. 30ml). Sauté until tender.

5. Remove from the heat then add the tofu back in and stir in the pesto to warm.

6. Plate the warm rice and top with the pesto-coated tofu and vegetables.

Options:
If you're not keen on sprouts or broccoli, swap for vegetables of choice.

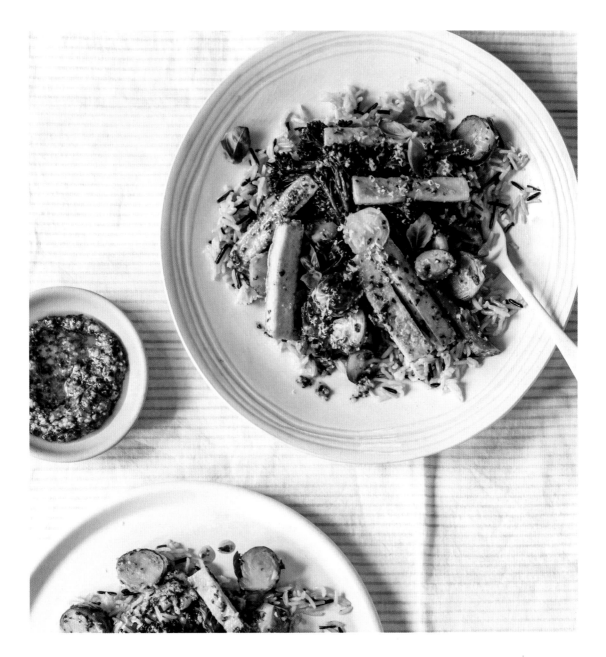

◆ In terms of health benefits, extra virgin olive oil (EVOO) is hands down the superior oil option. Loaded with polyphenols and other phytochemicals, the broad-ranging health benefits, including heart, brain and gut health, are supported by several trials. You can also cook with it, despite the myths. High-quality EVOO has a high smoking point (around 200°C) and research has shown that it's comparatively stable during home cooking, thanks to its high-antioxidant capacity, which protects the fat.

Korean BBQ squash taco shells with kimchi

A showcase of fermented food flavours – just another reason to be grateful for our microbial friends. Both gochujang, a fermented red chilli paste, and kimchi, a fermented side dish, have exploded in popularity in recent years, owing to the winning combination of flavours and attributed health benefits. Offering close to 10 grams of fibre per portion, this is one dish you have to try!

Base:
1 medium butternut squash, peeled and quartered (approx. 750g)
3 cloves of garlic, minced
3 spring onions, sliced
2 tbsp tamari or soy sauce
1 tbsp sesame oil
1 Medjool date, made into a paste with 1 tbsp boiling water using the back of a spoon
1½ tbsp gochujang
a twist of pepper
8 mini seeded tortillas (or fermented wrap on page 273)

Toppers:
2 tomatoes, diced
50g kimchi (see page 270)
60g live thick yoghurt (see page 280)
1 avocado, sliced
a handful of chopped coriander
2 tbsp sesame seeds (optional)

1. Preheat the oven to 170°C fan/375°F/gas mark 5.

2. Grate the squash, using a food processor or hand grater.

3. Place all the base ingredients, except for the squash, into a large bowl and mix well. Stir in the grated squash, making sure everything is coated. Leave to marinate for 20 minutes while you prepare the toppers and try the 'do nothing' exercise (see page 168).

4. Place the marinated squash on a baking tray. Place in the oven and bake for 15 minutes before giving it a quick mix. Place back in the oven for a further 5 minutes, or until caramelized on the outside.

5. Meanwhile, place a baking rack over a baking pan and hang each tortilla upside down on the rack. Place in the oven, with the squash, for the final 10–15 minutes.

6. Allow the tortilla shells to cool before filling with a spoonful of warm Korean BBQ squash then top with all the good stuff: tomatoes, kimchi, yoghurt, avocado, coriander, and sesame seeds, if using.

Options:
• Short on time? Steam the squash in the microwave for 5 minutes before coating in the marinade and browning in the oven for a final 10 minutes.
• Want to really impress your friends? Replace the squash with jackfruit.
• Sensitive to spicy food? Halve the quantity of gochujang, which is available online, or in most Asian grocers.

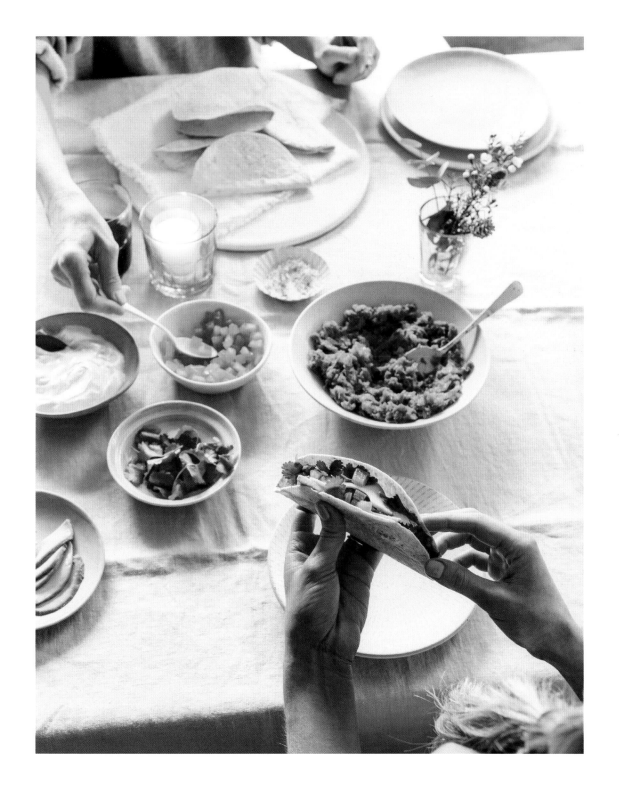

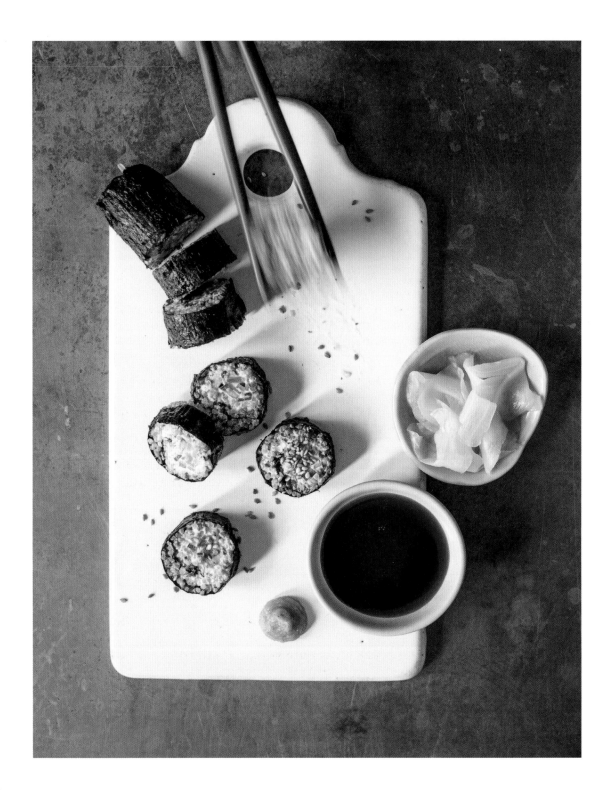

Quinoa sushi rolls

Offering double the fibre of shop-bought sushi, this is a high-protein fibre-boosted tweak on my childhood favourite. I also added in red onion, which is an especially good source of the polyphenol quercetin, known for its antioxidant benefits.

Base:
1 tsp miso paste
1 tbsp flaxseed, milled
120g quinoa, cooked
2 sheets nori (seaweed)

Toppers:
30g live thick yoghurt
  (see page 280)
½ a carrot, julienned (cut
  into matchsticks) or
  sliced into sheets
½ a cucumber, julienned
½ a red pepper, julienned
⅛ a red onion,
  julienned
½ an avocado, sliced into
  strips
60g smoked salmon (or
  protein of choice)

Extras:
pickled ginger or
  raw-slaw (see page 268)
light soy sauce, or
  dipping sauce of choice

1. Place the miso, flaxseed and 1 tablespoon of hot water into a small mug and combine, then pour it over the quinoa and stir through. Place in the fridge for 10 minutes to thicken while you prepare the toppers.

2. Cover your bamboo roller (or folded kitchen cloth) with a large piece of cling film. Place a nori sheet on top of the mat and spread half a cup (60g) of quinoa across three-quarters of the nori sheet. Leave a quarter of the nori roll free to help seal it (step 5). Press the quinoa firmly into the mat using the bottom of a cup.

3. Across the quinoa, 5cm from the edge, spread 2 tablespoons of yoghurt.

4. Lay the strips of carrot, cucumber, pepper, onion, avocado and salmon, if using, on top of the yoghurt.

5. To roll, start with the edge closest to the filling. Tightly roll the end over the filling, pressing as you go. Press the edges together at the end, using a tiny bit of water on the sheet's edge to help seal it.

6. With a sharp knife, cut into pieces and serve with pickles and a dipping sauce.

Options:
• Try replacing the cucumber with sugar snap peas and sprinkle the quinoa with sesame seeds.
• The topper options are endless – experiment with your favourite flavours.

◆ *Regular consumption of seaweed has been shown to modify your GM's genetic potential, meaning they develop the ability to digest parts of the seaweed. This is something that an untrained GM can't do. What does that mean for you? A GM with more skills: sign me up!*

Dinner

No matter what sort of day you've had, I'm a firm believer that dinner shouldn't add to your worries. If you're after convenience, you'll find the 'mix-and-match' gut-goodness bowls, which are all about laying down the foundation for a DIY throw-together dish that doesn't fall short on taste or diversity. For those Friday-night cravings, you'll find pizza duos and a spicy beanburger with options to match everyone's nutritional needs and flavour requests. What about the meat-lovers? Even they'll be singing your praises between the meatless meatballs in rich tomato sauce and the meaty lentil and mushroom fettuccine.

A bowl of butterbean curry

This rich, creamy curry, served in an edible bowl of roasted butternut, really does symbolize the idea of 'comfort in a bowl'. It's also loaded with vitamins A, K and C, making it quite a nourishing bowl. Short on time? Don't let that put you off. Ditch the edible bowl and just go with the curry – it's one of my winter staples.

Base (optional butternut bowl):

2 small butternut squash, halved lengthways and deseeded (approx. 900g)
1 tsp olive oil

Toppers (the curry):

2 tsp olive oil
½ an onion, chopped finely
1 clove of garlic, sliced
10g ginger, grated
2 tbsp Thai red curry paste
1 tsp curry powder
200g tinned chopped tomatoes
400g tinned coconut milk
400g tinned butterbeans, rinsed and drained
400g butternut squash, cooked
80–150g leafy greens of choice (I love bokchoy and spinach)
200g boneless white fish of choice (optional)
2 tbsp tamari (or soy sauce)
100g frozen peas
15g fresh coriander, finely chopped
lime juice, fresh, to taste

Butternut bowl (optional)

1. Preheat the oven to 190°C fan/400°F/gas mark 6.

2. Place the butternut squash in a microwave-safe dish with a little water in the bottom, put the lid on and cook on high for 15 minutes, or until soft. Allow to cool before scooping out the flesh with a spoon, leaving a 2cm-thick rimmed butternut 'bowl'. Set the flesh aside for the curry.

3. Place the squash bowls on a lined baking tray and massage the olive oil into the flesh and skin. Bake for 20 minutes, or until golden brown.

The curry

1. Place a large frying pan over a high heat, add the olive oil, onion, garlic, ginger, Thai curry paste and curry powder and stir for 2–3 minutes, or until fragrant.

2. Add the chopped tomatoes, coconut milk, butterbeans and the butternut squash flesh. Reduce the heat to a gentle simmer for 10–15 minutes.

3. Add your leafy greens (and fish, if using) and continue stirring for 3 minutes, or until the greens (and fish) are almost cooked.

4. Add the tamari, frozen peas and coriander. Taste and adjust the flavours to your preference. Once the peas are cooked and the greens still have a little bit of crunch to them, turn the heat off.

5. Squeeze in lime juice to taste, spoon into the baked butternut case (or any bowl) and serve warm.

◆ *The claims around ginger being a remedy for indigestion and nausea are backed by science. How? Trials have shown that ginger, albeit at fairly high doses, can speed up the emptying of food from your stomach into your small intestine.*

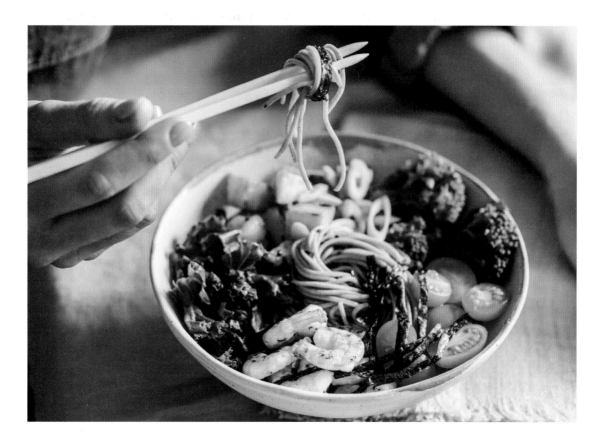

Serves 1

Mix-and-match gut-goodness bowls

Select one column of ingredients or create your own combo by picking one ingredient per row.

1. Cook the items as described. Grill foods with a drizzle of olive oil. Prepare your grains according to packet instructions. Steam in a pot or microwave.

2. Combine 'dress and coat' ingredients.

3. Assemble your bowl and finish with a dress and coat.

	Monday	Tuesday	Wednesday	Thursday	Friday
Fibre base (approx. 2 cups raw)	Peas Cauliflower (*steamed*)	Sweet potato (*steamed*) Onion (*sliced and fried*)	Kale (*steamed*)	Broccoli (*steamed*) Sugar snap peas	Courgette ribbons (*grilled*)
Golden grains (80–120g cooked)	Wild or brown rice	Soba (buckwheat) noodles	Quinoa	Wheat berries	Wholegrain pasta (*of choice*)
Polyphenol hit (½ cup) (keep raw)	Red pepper Coriander (1 tbsp)	Baby spinach	Sweetcorn	1 seaweed sheet (*torn into strips*)	Cherry tomatoes
Fermented flavours (1–2 tbsp)	Kimchi (page 270)	Raw-slaw (page 268)	Live thick yoghurt (page 280)	Pickles (page 219)	Shaved Parmesan
Prebiotic boost (to taste)	Banana (*sliced*)	Asparagus (*grilled*)	Chopped spring onion (*raw*)	Savoy cabbage	Brussels sprouts (*grilled*)
Healthy fats (1 tbsp)	Cashews	Pumpkin seeds	Avocado	Sesame seeds	Walnuts
Protein punch (80–120g)	Chicken breast	Tofu (*firm*)	Two eggs (*boiled or fried*)	Seafood of choice (*mackerel, salmon, prawns, squid*)	White legume (e.g. butter-beans) (*rinsed, drained and warmed*)
Dress and coat (1–2 tbsp) (adjust to taste, including a pinch of salt)	**Red curry** Thai red curry paste (2 tsp)* Live yoghurt (¼ cup, 60g) Desiccated coconut (2 tsp)	**Wholegrain Mustard** Wholegrain mustard (1 tsp) Olive oil (½ tbsp)	**Hot sauce** Sriracha hot sauce (½ tsp) Minced ginger (1 tsp) Cider vinegar (½ tsp)	**Miso sauce** White miso paste (1 tsp) Live yoghurt (¼ cup, 60g)	**Basil dressing** Extra virgin olive oil (½ tbsp) Lemon juice (1 tsp) 4 basil leaves (*finely chopped*)

*Use this to coat the protein, along with a brush of olive oil, before grilling.

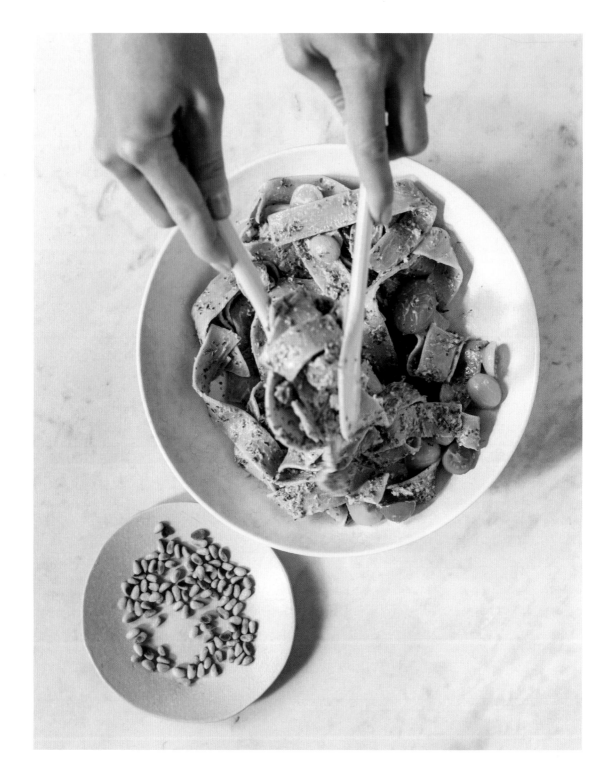

Creamy pistachio and spinach pesto pasta

For those nightmare days when all you want is something quick and tasty. And don't worry, it's got your microbes covered, too, with the prebiotic pistachios and 9 grams of fibre per portion – it's a real GM favourite.

Base:
200g wholegrain pasta of choice

Topper (pesto):
80g spinach leaves
20g basil leaves, fresh
65g pistachios
½ an avocado
2 tsp lemon juice, fresh
1 clove of garlic
3 tbsp nutritional yeast
2 tbsp extra virgin olive oil
100g live thick yoghurt (see page 280)
a pinch of salt, or to taste

Extras:
1 punnet cherry tomatoes, halved (approx. 300g)
2 tbsp pine nuts (optional)
cracked pepper, to taste

1. Place all the pesto ingredients into a blender along with 2 tablespoons of water. Blitz roughly to your preferred texture. You may need to scrape any mixture that has risen up the sides a few times.

2. Cook the pasta according to the packet instructions, then coat with the pesto sauce and leave for 5 minutes to infuse.

3. Serve topped with cherry tomatoes and pine nuts, if using, and some cracked pepper.

Options:
• Replace the nutritional yeast with 35g freshly grated Romano or Parmesan cheese.

◆ *It's worth paying a bit extra for extra virgin olive oil. Making EVOO is an expensive process. While a higher price doesn't always ensure quality, the cheapest bottle on the shelf is unlikely to be the real thing. To save on cost, I buy in bulk and decant a portion into a dark bottle (which protects it from the light), as I use it in all my cooking.*

Satay tofu skewers bedded with a side of saucy greens

I grew up in Queensland, where al fresco dining happens all year round. These skewers remind me of home, of sitting around the table watching them sizzle away on the barbecue. Sided with chewy grains and tender greens, this dish is high in protein and will bring you half your daily fibre needs.

YOU WILL NEED A PACKET OF SKEWERS.

Toppers:
3 tbsp Sriracha or chilli sauce
2 tbsp tamari
1 tbsp sesame oil
½ a Medjool date, softened, or sweetener of choice
5g peanut butter
½ tsp garlic powder
firm tofu, sliced into 4cm cubes (approx. 280g)
1 red and 1 yellow pepper, sliced into 4cm squares

Base:
1 tsp sesame oil
2 cloves of garlic, sliced
600g mixed greens, sliced
precooked wheat berries, or grain of choice (approx. 400g)
tamari, to taste
salt and pepper to taste

Dipping sauce:
live thick yoghurt (optional; see page 280)

1. Place all the toppers (apart from the tofu and peppers) into a large bowl and mix well. Stir in the tofu and leave to marinate for at least 1 hour.

2. Once marinated, skewer the tofu, alternating with the peppers. Set aside any leftover marinade.

3. Place on the BBQ or griddle pan on a moderate heat. Char on each side, then lower the heat and cook through, for approximately 2 minutes each side. Cover and take off the direct heat.

4. Place a large frying pan over a high heat and add the sesame oil and garlic. Cook for 1–2 minutes then add in the greens and wheat berries. Stir-fry for 2–3 minutes, or until the greens have wilted. Take off the heat, drizzle on the tamari and season to taste.

5. Serve the stir-fry topped with the skewers and a side of remaining marinade for dipping.

Options:
• Try replacing the grains with lentils for a higher prebiotic punch.
• Short on time? Replace the topper flavours with 70g peanut butter, 2 tsp curry powder and 100ml coconut milk.

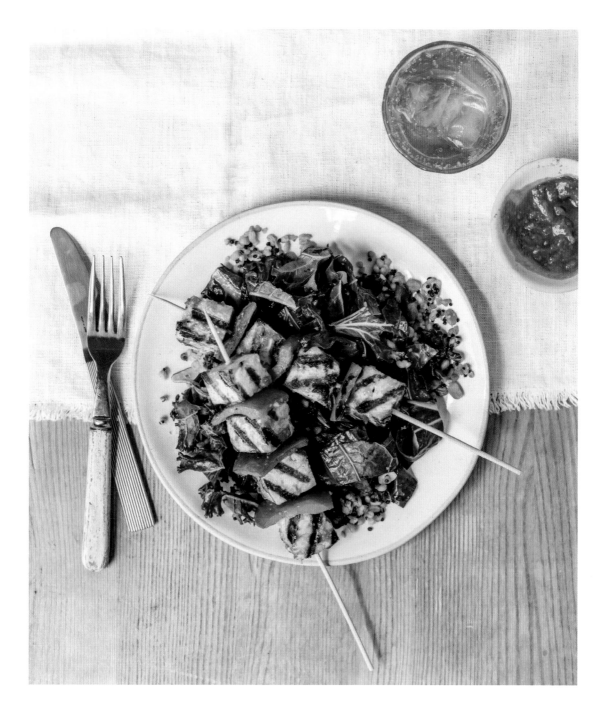

◆ *My first wheat berry experience was within weeks of moving to the UK, and it certainly was love at first bite. Their chewy texture, coupled with their subtle nut flavour, has earned them a regular place in my diet.*

Aubergine cannelloni with beetroot salsa and cashew cheese

After that wow factor? Then this dish is for you! The compliments won't stop on presentation – the creamy cashew cheese matched with the zesty salsa and succulent aubergine makes it one to remember.

Base:
2 aubergines (approx. 600g)

Toppers:
CASHEW CHEESE:
see recipe, page 213

BEETROOT SALSA:
400g packet of cooked beetroot in vinegar
8 cherry tomatoes
20g coriander leaves
2 tsp lemon juice, fresh
1 tsp chilli flakes
2 tbsp extra virgin olive oil
salt and pepper to taste

OLIVE PESTO:
30g feta cheese, crumbled
2 tbsp extra virgin olive oil
45g Kalamata black olives, pitted
115g tinned cannellini beans, rinsed and drained

1. Preheat the oven to 170°C fan/375°F/gas mark 5.

2. Slice the aubergine lengthways into thin sheets (approx. 1cm thick).

3. Grease a griddle pan and put it on a medium to high heat, then add the aubergine and grill for 5 minutes on each side, or until cooked through.

4. Meanwhile, place all the cashew cheese ingredients in a blender and blend until smooth.

5. Rinse the blender with water, then place all the beetroot salsa ingredients into it. Combine roughly and set aside.

6. Rinse the blender with water again, then place all the olive pesto ingredients into it and blend to a coarse consistency.

7. Lay out the grilled aubergine strips, layer each one with cashew cheese then the olive pesto, topped with a little salsa, roll up, and place them in a greased ovenproof dish.

8. Bake in the oven for 15 minutes, or until the flavours have cooked through and the tops are golden brown.

9. To serve, spread a spoonful of beetroot salsa on each plate and add the stuffed cannelloni. Top the cannelloni with a little more salsa.

Options:
• Serve with coriander leaves.

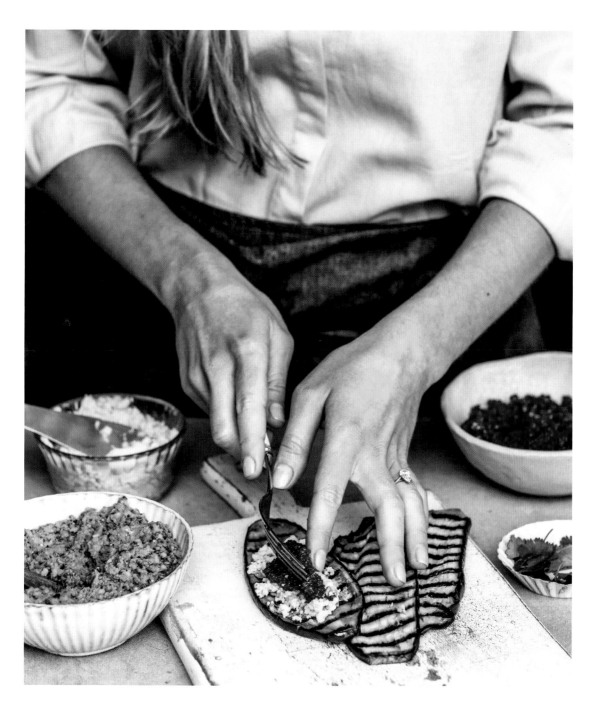

◆ *Beetroot is a great source of nitrate, which is considered Mother Nature's alternative to blood-pressure-lowering medications. In fact, there are several trials showing a benefit in people with high blood pressure.*

Pizza duo

It's all about the base – thin and crispy. Pizza is such a fun, versatile meal and it can be easily adapted to accommodate both your and your microbes' nutritional needs and taste preferences – it's one that everyone can enjoy. Here are two of my favourites, boasting over 10g of fibre per portion.

Spelt and quinoa

Base:
120g wholemeal spelt flour (additional for kneading)
1 tsp mixed Italian herbs
2 tsp baking powder
a pinch of salt
50g quinoa, cooked
110g thick Greek yoghurt
½ tbsp extra virgin olive oil

Pizza sauce:
150g cherry tomatoes
2 tbsp chopped basil
6 sundried tomato halves, preserved in oil
1 clove of garlic
1 tbsp olive oil

Topping inspo:
(Pick one or add your own favourites)
• sautéed mushrooms, spinach
• leaves and goat's cheese
• roast peppers, rocket and pine nuts,
• Kalamata olives, grilled artichoke hearts and ricotta cheese

1. Preheat the oven to 180°C fan/400°F/gas mark 6.

2. In a large bowl, combine the dry base ingredients (flour, herbs, baking powder and salt), then stir in the quinoa and fold in the yoghurt. Using your hands, form a wet dough. Knead on a floured surface for 3–4 minutes, rolling into balls, then flattening out (think of it as yoga for your pizza dough). Separate into two balls before placing in a bowl and coating with the oil. Cover with an inverted bowl and leave to sit somewhere warm for 15 minutes, while you prep the toppings.

3. Place all the pizza sauce ingredients into a blender and mix roughly.

4. Place the rested dough on a clean work surface and, using your hands, spread out to form your pizza base. Pinch the edge to form a crust.

5. Bake for 10 minutes, or until slightly golden, ideally on a tray with holes in the bottom so the pizza base gets nice and crispy.

6. Once the base is cooked, spread with the pizza sauce and add additional toppings. Bake for a further 5–10 minutes, depending on your choice of topping.

7. Slice and serve.

Options:
• Prefer to keep your hands clean? Use a wholegrain wrap as your base (see page 247). Replace the spices with fresh herbs of your choice, for example, oregano or basil.

Buckwheat and oat

Short on time? No oven required for this base, it's a simple case of 5 minutes in the frying pan and your low-FODMAP pizza is ready.

Base:
½ tbsp olive oil
  (additional for frying)
70g buckwheat
40g rolled oats
1 large egg
a pinch of salt
1 tsp baking powder

Pizza sauce (low-FODMAP):
150g cherry tomatoes
2 tbsp chopped basil
6 sundried tomato halves,
  preserved in oil
1 tbsp garlic-infused
  olive oil

Topping inspo:
(Pick one or add
your own favourites)
• hummus (see page
  240), chargrilled
  peppers and plum
  tomatoes
• ricotta spread,
  roasted butternut and
  caramelized red onion
• tahini dressing (see page
  232), smoked salmon,
  spinach and sauerkraut

Low-FODMAP
topping inspo:
• roast aubergine, green
  olives and feta
• BBQ chicken, roasted
  peppers and mozzarella
• Kalamata olives,
  Parmesan and rocket

1. Put all the base ingredients into a blender along with 200ml of water and blitz for 30 seconds.

2. Warm a little oil in a non-stick frying pan over a medium heat. Pour one-third of a cup (75ml) of the batter into the pan to form a mini pizza.

3. Cook for approximately 3 minutes, until there are bubbles in the base and you can lift it to flip easily.

4. Once flipped, turn the heat down and add on the sauce and toppings of choice. Place a lid or another pan over the top to seal in the heat. Repeat with the remaining batter.

Chargrilled miso aubergine with sweet potato wedges

Serves 2

A meaty dish that marries a succulent fillet of marinated aubergine with crispy-skinned potato wedges. This high-fibre dish wouldn't be complete without the creamy tahini dressing, which is so tasty I always make a double batch for my gut-goodness bowls.

Base:
olive oil for grilling
1 large aubergine, cut into 4 fillets lengthways

Toppers:
MISO MARINADE:
1½ tbsp miso paste
1 clove of garlic, crushed
2 tsp sesame oil
½ a Medjool date, stirred into a paste with 1 tbsp hot water

TAHINI DRESSING:
1 tbsp tahini
1 tbsp extra virgin olive oil
juice of ½ a lemon
½ a clove of garlic, crushed
salt and pepper, to taste

ROASTED VEGETABLES:
1 large sweet potato, cut into thin wedges (approx. 300g)
2 tsp olive oil
150g cherry tomatoes
salt and pepper to taste

Extras:
side salad of rocket or leaves of choice

1. Preheat the oven to 170°C fan/375°F/gas mark 5.

2. Place an oiled griddle pan on a high heat and chargrill the aubergine for 2 minutes on each side, or until brown char lines are formed. (If you're short on time, skip this step.)

3. Place the miso marinade ingredients with 1 tablespoon of water into a small bowl and combine.

4. Place the tahini dressing ingredients into another small bowl with 1 tablespoon of water and combine.

5. Transfer the aubergine to an oven tray lined with baking paper and pour over the miso marinade. Using your hands, massage into the flesh and bake in the oven for 10 minutes.

6. Place the sweet potato wedges in a microwave-safe dish with a little water in the bottom, put the lid on and cook on high for 4 minutes to soften.

7. Pat the wedges dry then toss in oil with the tomatoes and sprinkle with seasoning.

8. Turn up the oven to 170°C fan/375°F/gas mark 5, add the wedges and tomatoes to the aubergine and cook for a further 15–20 minutes, or until crisp on the outside.

9. Serve the aubergine fillets alongside the wedges, tomatoes and rocket, or leaves of choice. Drizzle with the tahini dressing before diving in.

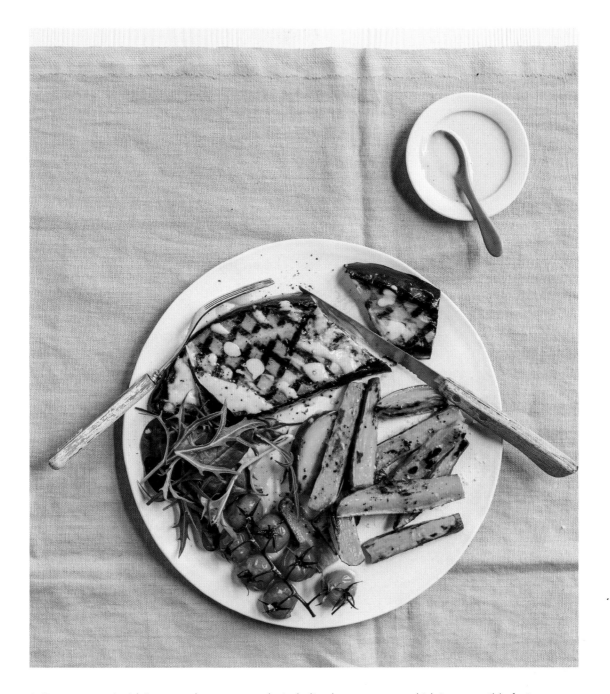

◆ *Sweet potato is rich in many plant compounds, including beta-carotene, which is responsible for its orange glow. This antioxidant is transformed into vitamin A in our body to support immunity and eye health. To maximize the beta-carotene absorption, I've added olive oil – the resulting crispy crunch is a bonus.*

Meatless meatballs in rich tomato sauce

I might be a little biased, but my microbes and I much prefer these to the meat version – they're incredibly tender, full of flavour and provide 15 grams of fibre per portion.

Base:
1 tbsp olive oil
1 aubergine, diced (approx. 400g)
1 onion, chopped
1 tsp garlic powder
35g Kalamata olives, sliced
3 sundried tomatoes, preserved in oil
2 tbsp Worcestershire sauce
2 tsp mixed Italian herbs
a pinch of salt
10g fresh basil
2 tbsp flaxseed, milled
60g rolled oats

Toppers:
TOMATO SAUCE:
1 tsp olive oil
1 clove of garlic
3 sundried tomato halves, preserved in oil
200g tinned chopped tomatoes
2 tbsp basil, chopped
a pinch of salt

Optional:
live thick yoghurt (see page 280) or Parmesan
40g spinach leaves

1. Preheat the oven to 170°C fan/375°F/gas mark 5.

2. Place a large frying pan over a medium heat, add the olive oil and all the base ingredients (apart from the basil, flax and oats) and sauté for 5–10 minutes, or until starting to colour.

3. Place the flax and oats into a food processor and blend to form coarse crumbs. Place in a bowl and set aside. Place the sautéed mix, along with the basil, into the food processor. Combine roughly.

4. Stir the sautéed mix into the crumb mixture and leave in the fridge to thicken for 10 minutes.

5. Once chilled, roll into 'meatballs' (makes around 12, of approx. 40g each) and place on an oven tray lined with baking paper, then place in the oven for 20 minutes, or until golden brown.

6. Meanwhile, prepare your tomato sauce. Place a saucepan over a medium heat and add the oil, garlic and sundried tomatoes. Fry for a few minutes, then add in the remaining ingredients. Reduce the heat to a gentle simmer for approx. 20 minutes, stirring every few minutes.

7. Serve the meatballs on a bed of spinach topped with tomato sauce and a dollop of yoghurt or Parmesan.

Options:
- Spice things up with half a chilli.
- For vegans: Replace the Worcestershire sauce with barbecue sauce and omit the yoghurt and cheese for serving.

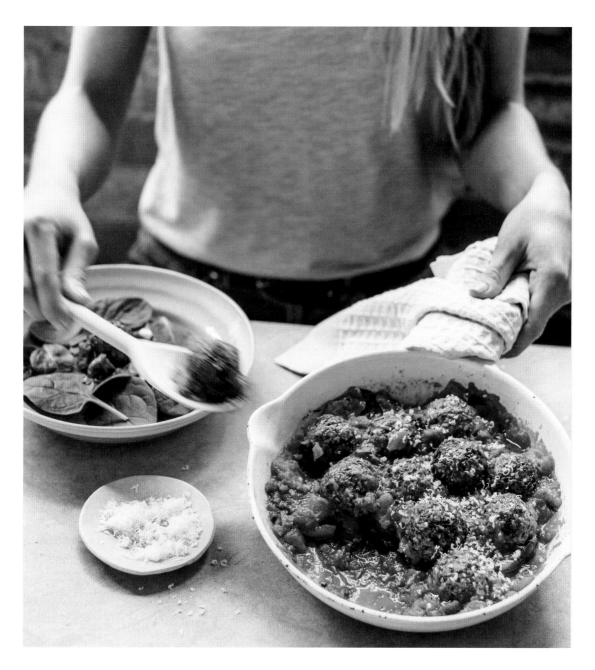

◆ *Garlic has been used for its medicinal benefits for thousands of years, and now we have the science to back it up. Although most of the benefits from trials on blood pressure and cholesterol management use high-dose supplements, regularly including garlic in your diet can only help. What about its flu-fighting power? There have been some placebo-controlled trials (meaning good quality) to support this too.*

Spicy bean burgers

BBQs just got a whole lot tastier with these burgers. Combining the prebiotic goodness of the legumes and polyphenols from the herbs and spices, the burger alone offers over 5 grams of fibre, making it a tasty feast for your microbes too.

Base:
130g sweet potato, chopped
1 x 400g tin of mixed beans, drained and rinsed
1 spring onion, chopped
60g carrot, grated
1 large egg
1 tsp garlic powder
1 tsp cumin
10g fresh coriander, chopped
1 tsp smoked paprika
1 tsp chilli (fresh or flakes)
1 tbsp soy sauce
1 tbsp lime juice, fresh
a twist of black pepper
40g rolled oats
1 tsp arrowroot
50g cheese (optional)

Toppers:
BURGER COATING:
40g desiccated coconut

CARAMELIZED ONIONS:
1 red onion, cut into ½cm-thick rings
½ a Medjool date, diced
1 tbsp balsamic vinegar
1 tbsp olive oil

Extras:
wholegrain burger bun (or go naked)
pickled beetroot, sliced
tomatoes, sliced
live thick yoghurt

1. Place the sweet potato and a small splash of water into a microwave-safe dish. Cover and cook on high for 4 minutes. Drain and cool.

2. Place the beans, spring onion and carrot into a large bowl and mix together. Set aside approx. 1 cup (130g) and place the rest in a food processor.

3. Place the remaining base ingredients, apart from the oats, arrowroot and cheese, in a food processor. Blend roughly.

4. Stir in the oats, arrowroot, cheese (if using) and reserved bean mix from step 2 and place in the fridge for 10 minutes, to firm up.

5. Place the caramelized onion ingredients into a small saucepan with 80ml of water and cook on a low heat for 15–20 minutes, or until soft and caramelized.

6. Roll the chilled mix into burgers (approx. 75g) and gently coat with coconut.

7. Place a frying pan with olive oil over a low–medium heat. Add the burgers and cook for 4–5 minutes on each side, or until golden brown.

8. Finally, the burger build! Layer the bun with the beetroot, tomatoes, a dollop of yoghurt, if using, followed by the burger and caramelized onions.

Options:
• Have some leftover dip from pages 240–42? Add a dollop to your burger.

◆ *Cumin is packed full of plant bioactives that are linked to improved immunity, heart health and even digestion – this ancient spice is not just a tasty addition.*

Serves 4

Lentil and mushroom fettuccine

My favourite dish growing up was my Nanna's traditional fettuccine, which, although it was oh so tasty, didn't provide much goodness for my microbes. I challenged myself to make a meat-free version, with all the flavour but none of the meat. Turned out to be quite the hit – the family didn't miss the meat either. And it delivers over 50 per cent of our daily fibre recommendations per portion.

Base:
200g wholegrain
  fettuccine of choice

Toppers:
1 onion, chopped
2 cloves of garlic,
  chopped
1 stick of celery, chopped
1 carrot, chopped
1 courgette, chopped
1 red pepper, chopped
150g mushrooms,
  chopped
2 tbsp olive oil
3 bay leaves
1 tsp mixed Italian herbs
1 x 400g tin of green
  lentils, drained and
  rinsed
1 x 400g tin of tomatoes
6 sundried tomato halves,
  preserved in oil, chopped
2 tbsp tomato paste
2 tbsp capers
400ml vegetable stock
salt and pepper to taste

To serve:
Parmesan cheese or
  nutritional yeast

1. Place all the fresh vegetables (onion, garlic, celery, carrot, courgette, pepper, mushrooms) into a blender, and blitz for a few seconds until finely chopped.

2. Place a large saucepan over a medium heat and add the olive oil, bay leaves, herbs and chopped vegetables. Sauté for 10 minutes, or until the water has evaporated.

3. Stir the lentils, tinned and sundried tomatoes and tomato paste, capers and vegetable stock into the sautéed vegetables. Season to taste and reduce to a gentle simmer for 25 minutes, with the lid off, to allow the liquid to evaporate, stirring occasionally. Remove the bay leaves.

4. Ten minutes before the sauce is ready (it should be thickening up and rich in flavour), cook the fettucine al dente according to the packet instructions (approximately 10–12 minutes).

5. Drain the pasta and stir in the sauce. Leave to sit for a few minutes, then grate some Parmesan or sprinkle nutritional yeast over it and serve.

◆ *Not ready to part with all your mince? Meet me halfway – 50 per cent mince, 50 per cent lentils – and you'll have a tasty meal which is responsible for almost 50 per cent less greenhouse gas emissions.*

Snacks

Whether you consider yourself a snacker or not, these recipes will get you thinking a little differently about these hunger quenchers. Although snacks are notorious for neglecting the needs of our GM (low in fibre and high in added sugar and salt) and being problematic for those with food intolerances, it certainly doesn't have to be that way. In the pages to follow you'll find plenty to inspire your savoury snacking needs, each with a gut-health twist.

Sweet snacks can be a real mood-booster. But imagine ones that don't just lift your mood but the mood of your GM too. Well, imagine no more, because this is what my sweet snacks are all about! Whether you're looking for that 3 p.m. pick-me-up, a movie-night treat, or a snack to pull out when you're looking to turn some heads, I've got you covered.

Sesame and kale crisps

You'll never look at kale the same way again. A game-changer for all those who are anti-greens, it makes the perfect after-work snack or TV-time accompaniment.

Base:

125g kale, destalked and
   chopped into pieces

Toppers:

1 tsp tahini
1 tsp garlic powder
1 tbsp olive oil
a pinch of sea salt
1 tbsp sesame seeds

1. Preheat the oven to 160°C fan/350°F/gas mark 4.

2. Place the tahini, garlic, oil and salt into a large bowl and stir. Once combined, add the kale, and toss to evenly coat the kale bites. Sprinkle with sesame seeds.

3. On two lined baking trays, spread out the kale leaves, minimizing overlap. Bake for 10 minutes, or until crisp, flip, and repeat on the other side for an additional 5 or so minutes. Keep a close eye on the crisps and remove any that start to brown.

4. Allow to cool before tucking in.

Options:

• Add a teaspoon of a herb of your choice.
• Replace the garlic powder and olive oil with garlic-infused olive oil to make this snack low-FODMAP.

Trio of dips

In terms of nutrition, dips have been given a pretty bad rap. While, for many shop-bought varieties, this may be warranted, don't let this taint your perception of home-made dips, which are one of my fridge essentials. Their use goes way beyond dipping. I use them as spreads, dressings, sauces, fillings – I add them to just about anything. They can transform any boring salad or bowl of veg, and they make a great afternoon snack when paired with veggie sticks or seeded crackers. Better still, these recipes are foolproof – add, blend, serve.

Hummus

Butter's prebiotic sibling, providing nourishment not just for you but your GM too.

Base:
400g tinned chickpeas,
   drained and rinsed
   (or use 240g cooked
   sprouted chickpeas; see
   page 278)
1 clove of garlic, crushed
1 tbsp tahini
60ml extra virgin olive oil
½ tsp cumin
½ tsp smoked paprika
2 tbsp lemon juice, fresh
a pinch of salt
a big twist of black
   pepper

Topper (optional):
pine nuts, toasted
   (pan-fry for 30 seconds,
   or until golden brown)
a shake of smoked
   paprika

1. Set aside 3 tbsp whole chickpeas for decoration.

2. Using a blender, blitz all the base ingredients with 60ml water until completely smooth (approx. 2 minutes). Taste as you go; you may like a little more lemon or salt.

3. Top the hummus with whole chickpeas and toasted pine nuts and/or paprika, if using.

Options:
• Tahini is crushed sesame seeds. Although available in most supermarkets, if you don't have any, you can replace it with unsalted peanut butter.

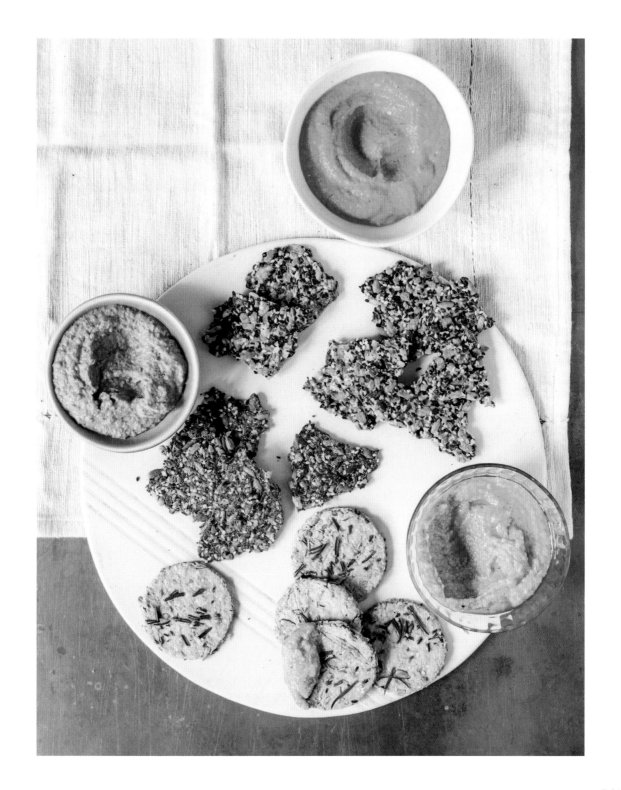

Pea and mint hummus

Creamy, minty – yum. Oh, and it's garlic- and onion-free, which is a rare find in the world of dips. While the peas still do provide some FODMAPs (they are prebiotic, after all), you can include a half-portion on the FODMAP-lite approach. It could also be a good one to test when going through the reintroduction stage (see page 152).

Base:
270g peas, defrosted
1 tsp tahini
2 tsp lemon juice, fresh
½ tsp cumin
2 tbsp olive oil
a pinch of salt
a handful of fresh mint
a twist of pepper

Toppers:
mixed seeds

1. Using a blender, blitz the peas, tahini, lemon juice, cumin, oil and salt with 60ml water until semi-smooth (1 minute).

2. Add the fresh mint and the pepper. Blend for a further minute, leaving a little of the texture from the mint leaves.

3. Serve topped with mixed seeds.

Harissa red pepper dip

Flavour-rich and nutrient-dense. The creamy hazelnuts have been shown to help manage our blood cholesterol, which is linked with lowering your risk of heart disease – flavour and health in one!

Base:
180g hazelnuts, toasted
  (or pan-fry for 2 minutes
  or until lightly brown)
1 tsp cumin seeds
360g jar of roasted
  peppers, drained
1 tsp honey, or sweetener
  of choice
1 tsp harissa
2 tsp lemon juice, fresh
a pinch of salt
a twist of black pepper

1. Set aside 5 or so whole hazelnuts for decoration.

2. Using a blender, blitz all the ingredients until they form a smooth paste (1 minute).

3. Serve topped with hazelnuts.

Trio of crackers

Another one of my pantry staples. They're packed with plant-based protein and healthy fats – I doubt you'll find another cracker that lives up to these specs. I make a batch of each and enjoy them on rotation.

Makes 12 oatcakes

Seedy oatcakes

You'll never want to buy oatcakes again. I tend to keep a stash of these in my bag to keep me going in between meals on those busy days.

Base:
80g rolled oats
40g mixed seeds
  (flaxseed, sunflower,
  pumpkin, sesame)
a pinch of salt
1 tbsp olive oil

Toppers (optional):
1 tsp rosemary, dried

1. Preheat the oven to 170°C fan/375°F/gas mark 5.

2. Place the oats in a blender and blitz to form coarse crumbs.

3. In a large bowl, place the oat crumbs, seeds and salt. Give it a quick stir, then mix in the oil and 60ml of warm water. Combine with your hands to form a wet dough. Leave to rest somewhere warm for 10 minutes, while you do some breathing (page 173) or pelvic-floor (page 184) exercise.

4. Line an oven tray with baking paper and place the dough in the middle. Place another sheet of baking paper on top of the dough and, using a rolling pin or a glass bottle, spread the dough into a thin layer – the thinner, the better.

5. Remove the top paper and sprinkle the rosemary over the dough, if using.

6. Using a cookie cutter (or a glass cup), cut out oatcake circles, pressing firmly to cut through the seeds, removing any excess dough.

7. Bake for 20–25 minutes, or until lightly brown.

Options:
Replace the rosemary with basil and black pepper.

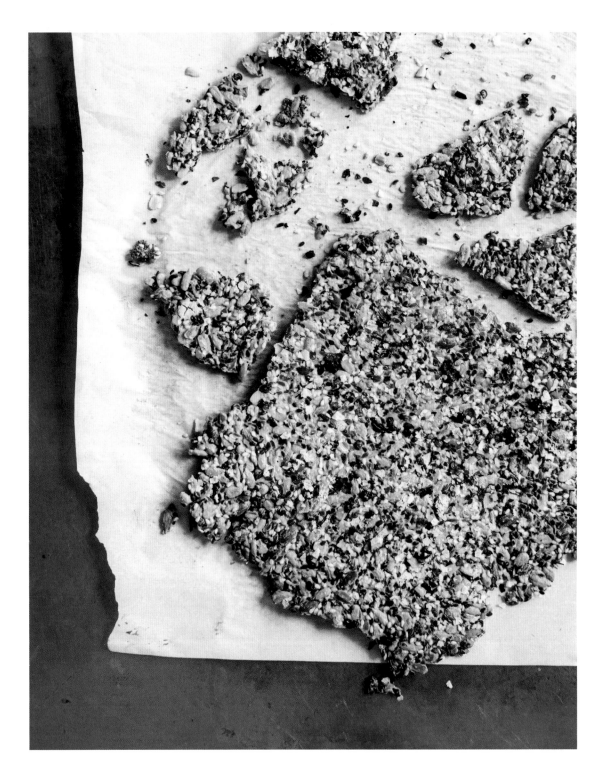

Cheesy vegan crackers

Gluten-free, dairy-free but not flavour-free. Oh, and they're low-FODMAP too.

Base:
35g buckwheat flour
25g ground flaxseeds
145g mixed seeds
  (flaxseed, sunflower,
  pumpkin, sesame)
20g poppy seeds
2 tbsp nutritional yeast
a pinch of salt
a big twist of pepper
2 tbsp olive oil

Toppers (optional):
½ tsp thyme
sea salt flakes

1. Preheat the oven to 160°C fan/350°F/gas mark 4.

2. In a large bowl, combine all the base ingredients together, apart from the oil.

3. Slowly pour in the oil and 75ml of hot water and, using your hands, make a wet dough. Leave to rest for 10 minutes somewhere warm.

4. Line an oven tray with baking paper and place the dough in the middle. Place another sheet of oven paper on top of the dough and, using a rolling pin or a glass bottle, spread the dough into a thin layer – the thinner, the better.

5. Remove the top paper and sprinkle the toppers, if using, over the dough and gently press in.

6. Bake for 25–30 minutes, or until slightly golden. Transfer to a cooling rack and when completely cool break into cracker size of choice.

Makes 20 small crackers

Spiced chickpea and sesame seed crackers

With a subtle hint of sesame seeds, this cracker is perfect for lifting any topping.

Base:
50g gram flour
145g mixed seeds
  (flaxseed, sunflower,
  pumpkin, sesame)
35g black sesame seeds
  (or white)
½ tsp cumin seeds
¼ tsp ground coriander
¼ tsp turmeric
a pinch of salt
a big twist of pepper
2 tbsp olive oil

Toppers (optional):
½ tsp chilli flakes
sea salt flakes

1. Repeat steps 1–5 of cheesy vegan crackers above.

2. Bake for 20–25 minutes, or until slightly golden.

3. Transfer to a cooling rack and when completely cool break into cracker size of choice.

Sea salt and rosemary legume crunch

Our favourite bar snack – the flavour and crunch for me, and the prebiotics and polyphenols for my microbes. These tasty treats offer close to 5 grams of plant-based protein making a great topper on any gut-goodness bowl (see page 222).

Base:
400g tinned 4-bean mix, or legume of choice, drained and rinsed
1 tbsp olive oil
2 tsp rosemary, dried
a pinch of salt

1. Preheat the oven to 180°C fan/400°F/gas mark 6.

2. Pat the legumes dry, then toss in a bowl with the olive oil and seasonings.

3. On a lined baking tray, spread out the legumes. Bake for 15–20 minutes, or until golden brown and crispy.

4. Allow to cool before tucking in.

Spelt wraps

It's near impossible to find an additive-free wrap on supermarket shelves (trust me, I've searched for one of my trials). So after playing around in the kitchen and discovering I could make them from scratch in less than five minutes, I've never looked back. I use this as my go-to base for the mix-and-match sliders (page 210).

Base:
65g wholemeal or
  wholemeal spelt flour
1 large egg
a pinch of salt

Topper (optional):
1 tsp sesame seeds

1. Place all the base ingredients into a bowl and whisk together with 120ml warm water for several minutes to form a fluffy, thin batter.

2. In a non-stick frying pan, warm a little oil over a medium heat. Add half a cup of the batter (120ml) to the pan and swirl around the bottom so you get an even wrap. Sprinkle with sesame seeds, if using.

3. Cook for approximately 1 minute, until there are bubbles in the wrap and you can lift it to flip easily.

4. Cook on the other side for a minute, or until slightly brown. Wrap in a clean tea towel to keep the moisture in until ready to serve.

◆ *Spelt is a good source of prebiotics. For those following a strict low-FODMAP diet, fermented spelt (aka sourdough) is considered low-FODMAP because microbes consume some of the FODMAPS.*

Coconut-crusted green dippers with a zesty dip

The humble green bean, all dressed up. This one is a real crowd-pleaser, particularly among my foodie friends. The crispy, coconutty dippers are brought to life with the zesty salsa dip, serving up a high-fibre, high-protein snack.

Base:
400g green beans

Toppers:
BATTER:
180ml milk of choice
30g coconut flour

CRUMB:
40g oats
25g desiccated coconut
½ tsp cumin seeds
½ tsp turmeric
½ tsp mustard seeds
2 tsp lime zest
a pinch of salt
a big twist of pepper
½ tsp chilli flakes
  (optional)

DIP:
240g live thick yoghurt
  (see page 280)
¼ a red onion, roughly
  sliced
1 tsp lime juice, fresh
a handful of coriander
a pinch of salt

1. Preheat the oven to 180°C fan/400°F/gas mark 6.

2. Using a blender, blitz the oats for a few seconds to form coarse crumbs.

3. Transfer the oats to a large bowl, add in all the other crumb ingredients and mix to combine.

4. Place the batter ingredients in a second bowl and mix. Leave to thicken for a few minutes.

5. Dip the beans into the batter (it will be quite thick so use your hands to help coat) and then into the crumb mix. Place on a lined baking tray.

6. Bake for 20 minutes, or until golden and crispy.

7. While the beans are baking, put all the dip ingredients together into a blender and blitz for a few seconds until roughly combined. Taste and adjust to preference. Serve alongside your crispy bean dippers.

Options:
For a low-FODMAP option, replace the onions with chives or the green end of spring onions and opt for a lactose-free yoghurt.

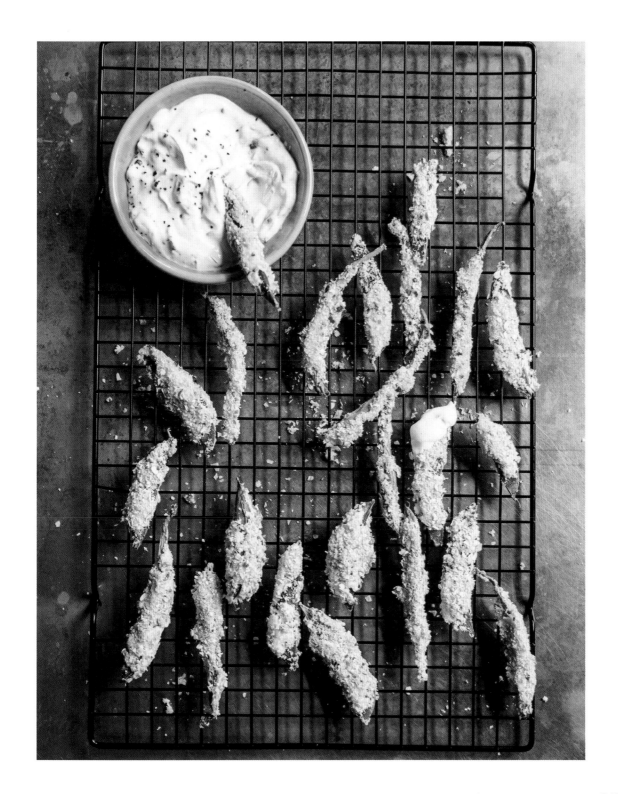

Sticky BBQ vegan wings

When your meat-loving brother asks for seconds, you know they must be good – finger-licking good. Unlike regular wings, these ones are not just feeding you but are also a feast for your GM. You'll also be treated to 10 grams of plant-based protein per portion.

Base:
2 tbsp self-raising flour
2 tbsp soy milk
1 head of cauliflower,
   cut into bite-size florets
100g almond meal
   (ground almonds)

Toppers:
170g ketchup
2 tsp soy sauce
2 tsp Worcestershire
   sauce (opt for anchovy-
   free, if vegan)
1 tsp smoked paprika
½ tsp garlic powder
1 tsp chipotle chilli flakes

1. Preheat the oven to 170°C fan/375°F/gas mark 5.

2. Place the flour and milk in a small bowl and combine to form a thin batter. Dry the cauliflower florets, then dunk into the batter. Shake off any excess then coat with the ground almonds.

3. Place on a lined baking tray and bake for 20 minutes, turning once. Meanwhile, in a small saucepan, combine all the topper ingredients and simmer for 2 minutes.

4. Remove the cauliflower from the oven and dip each floret into the mix in the saucepan. Return to the baking tray.

5. Turn the oven up to 170°C fan/375°F/gas mark 5 and bake the florets for a further 5–10 minutes, or until the 'wings' are crispy and the sauce has caramelized.

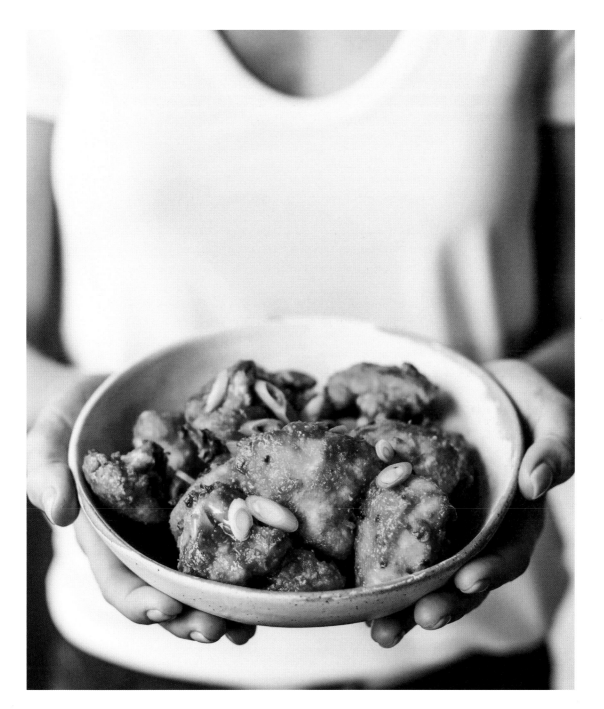

◆ *Plant chemicals found in cauliflower have been shown to directly support the health of the immune cells that line our intestine, at least in animal studies.*

Raw carrot cake balls

Makes 12 (25g each)

An indulgent treat that's also high in fibre and loaded with polyphenols – yes, it is possible. A single batch is never enough. Freeze in single portions and enjoy as a pre-gym snack or a mid-morning boost.

Base:
4 Medjool dates (approx. 60g pitted)
50g ground almonds
25g rolled oats
1 large carrot, grated (approx. 100g grated)
2 tbsp flaxseed, milled
1 tsp allspice
½ tsp cinnamon
1 tsp vanilla extract
15g coconut flakes
½ tsp ground ginger
1 tsp grated fresh ginger, if you like extra zing! (optional)

Topper:
FILLING
25g walnuts

COATING (optional)
(choose one)
desiccated coconut
poppy seeds
whole or ground linseeds
crushed nuts

1. Place the dates, almonds and oats into your food processor and blitz until everything is roughly blended.

2. Add the rest of the base ingredients and blitz again. The mixture should be moist but not so wet that you can't roll it (if it's too wet, add an extra sprinkle of oats).

3. Using a walnut half as the centre, form a ball around it with the mixture. Leave naked or roll in your coating of choice. Repeat.

4. Pop into the fridge to firm up for at least 2 hours.

Options:

• Can't get your hands on Medjool dates? Go for 60 grams of dried dates softened with water.
• Coat the balls with melted dark chocolate for an extra-indulgent treat.

◆ *A handful of walnuts a day for 3 weeks has been shown to increase microbes that produce the beneficial short-chain fatty acid butyrate. The walnuts also decreased specific compounds that are linked with colon cancer.*

Fudgy black bean brownies

I serve this tasty treat to all the fussy eaters in my life. Loaded with polyphenols and prebiotics, their microbes love me for it.

YOU WILL NEED CUPCAKE LINERS.

Base:
125g tinned black beans, drained and rinsed
2 large eggs
1 tsp vanilla extract
20g cocoa powder
80g rolled oats
1 tsp baking powder
8 small prunes (approx. 40g pitted)
6 Medjool dates (approx. 90g pitted)
1 large banana, extra-ripe (about 120g peeled weight)
120ml milk of choice
a pinch of salt
50g dark-chocolate chips
30g walnuts or 2 tbsp crunchy peanut butter (optional)

Topper:
live thick yoghurt (see page 280)
frozen berries
honey (optional)

1. Preheat the oven to 180°C fan/400°F/gas mark 6.

2. Place all the base ingredients, except the chocolate chips and nuts, if using, into a blender and blitz until completely smooth (around 3 minutes).

3. Place the cake liners into a bun or muffin tin, then spoon in the mix. Dot in the chocolate chips and nuts (if using).

4. Bake for 10–12 minutes, then allow to cool in the tin for 5 minutes. Best served warm along with a dollop of yoghurt (sweetened with honey, if using) and frozen berries of choice.

5. What about the leftovers? Wrap each portion individually and freeze. Next time you're craving a sweet snack, warm in the microwave before tucking in.

◆ *There is a convincing body of evidence to support the role of the polyphenols found in cocoa (flavanols) in lowering blood pressure, and also in improving clarity of thought as we age. Another study has shown that a single dose of a flavanol-rich chocolate drink (compared to flavanol-poor) counteracted the effects of sleep deprivation on memory in healthy women – sign me up!*

Cinnamon-spiced popcorn

Serves 2

When it comes to those afternoon sweet cravings, this high-fibre snack certainly hits the spot. Quick, easy, and oh so tasty.

YOU WILL NEED A
BROWN PAPER BAG.

50g popcorn kernels
1 tsp honey
¼ tsp cinnamon

1. Put the corn kernels into a brown paper bag and fold the top over twice to seal.

2. Microwave on high for approximately 3 minutes, or until you hear a pause of about 3 seconds between pops.

3. Leave to stand for 20 seconds, then carefully open the bag.

4. Drizzle in the honey, followed by the cinnamon. Reseal the bag and shake to combine.

Options:

- Experiment with other flavour combinations, such as olive oil (2 tsp), curry powder (½ tsp) and ground coriander (½ tsp) or vinegar (1 tsp) and salt (½ tsp).
- If you don't have a microwave, don't let that get between you and your hopes of cinnamon-spiced popcorn. Put a small amount of oil to coat the bottom of the biggest saucepan you have with a glass lid. Set it on a medium heat and put in a single layer of kernels before returning the lid. As soon as you see it beginning to pop, continuously shake the pan gently across the hob to ensure the kernels don't burn. After a minute or so, once the popping has slowed down significantly, remove from the heat. Allow it to cool briefly, then drizzle on the honey and cinnamon. Transfer to a bowl and tuck in.

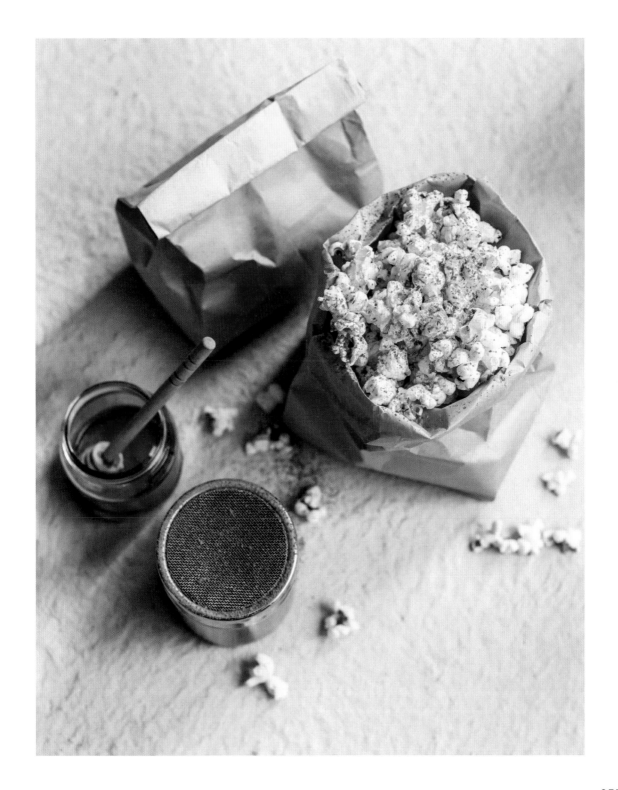

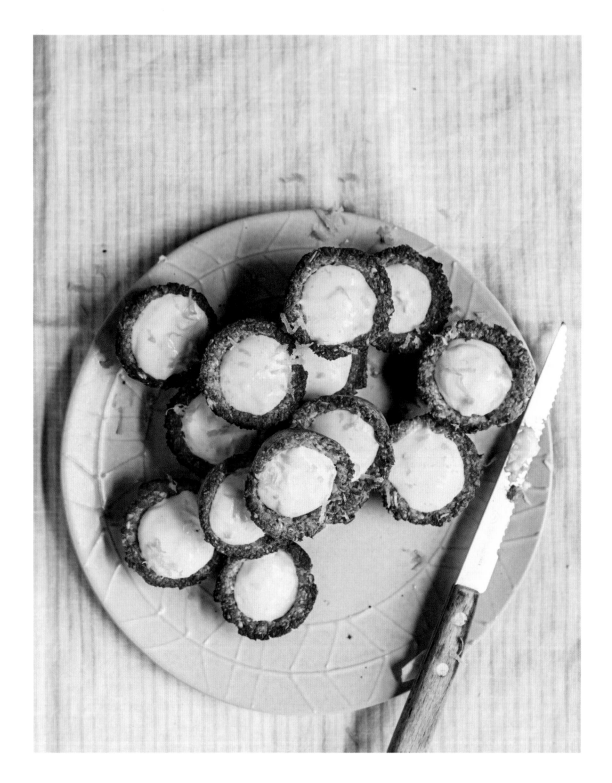

Lemon curd in chia and cashew tartlets

A gut-boosting twist on my favourite dessert – you'll find live microbes in the curd and prebiotics in the base. Beware: your GM may not let you stop at just one.

Base:
65g cashews
30g chia seeds
25g desiccated coconut
40g oats
4 Medjool dates (approx. 60g pitted), chopped

Topper:
70ml lemon juice (approx. 2 lemons)
1 tsp lemon zest (plus extra for garnishing)
3 tbsp honey, or sweetener of choice
10g arrowroot starch
170g live thick yoghurt (see page 280)

1. Preheat the oven to 140°C fan/320°F/gas mark 3.

2. Place all the base ingredients into a blender with 60ml of water and blitz until roughly combined. With your hands, roll the mix together to form a sticky dough and allow to rest for 10 minutes in the fridge.

3. While the dough is resting, grease mini-muffin tins with your oil of choice.

4. Once the dough has firmed up, press a tablespoonful (approx. 15g) into each mould. Use your fingertip to evenly spread the dough across the base and sides.

5. Bake for 15 minutes, or until golden brown. Set aside to cool.

6. Meanwhile, in a small saucepan over a low heat, combine the lemon juice, lemon zest, honey and arrowroot starch. Stir vigorously with a wooden spatula until the mix becomes a thick gel. Take off the heat and, once it has cooled a touch (1–2 minutes off the heat), stir in the yoghurt to form a spoonable mix. Taste as you go and adjust the lemon to taste.

7. Allow the tartlet cases to cool completely before dolloping the curd into each one. Refrigerate for at least 4 hours to set. Garnish with extra lemon zest.

Options:
- Prefer a crunchy tartlet case? Make the lemon curd first and allow to set, covered, in the fridge for 4 hours. Bake the cases and allow to cool. When ready to serve, dollop the thick curd into each case.
- Are you nut free? Replace the cashews with 40g of extra oats and one extra date.

Prebiotic chocolate bark

I always make these for my friends and family at Easter, wrapped up in tissue paper and tied with craft string – I'd hate for their microbes to feel left out of the celebrations.

Base:
200g good-quality white
    chocolate
2 tsp extra virgin olive oil
50g good-quality dark
    chocolate, 70% plus
    cocoa solids

Toppers:
50g dried mango,
    diced
50g crushed pistachios

1. Place the white chocolate in a small microwave-safe bowl and microwave for 40–60 seconds, stirring vigorously every 15 seconds, until melted.

2. To the melted white chocolate, add the oil, followed by half the toppers, and stir in. Pour the mixture on to a lined baking tray, thinly spreading the chocolate-coated mix and dotting in the rest of the toppers. Place in the fridge for 5 minutes to set.

3. Meanwhile, in a separate bowl, melt the dark chocolate in the microwave, as described above.

4. Once the white chocolate is firm, using a fork, drizzle on the dark chocolate with whipping movements. Place in the fridge for 30 minutes or until rock solid, then remove and break the bark into pieces.

◆ *The darker the chocolate, the higher the percentage of cocoa, which means the more polyphenols. This may explain why dark chocolate has been linked with decreased risk of heart disease and diabetes … albeit in moderation. In fact, one study found that daily consumption of cocoa, compared to a placebo group, significantly lowered participants' blood pressure – a key risk factor for heart disease.*

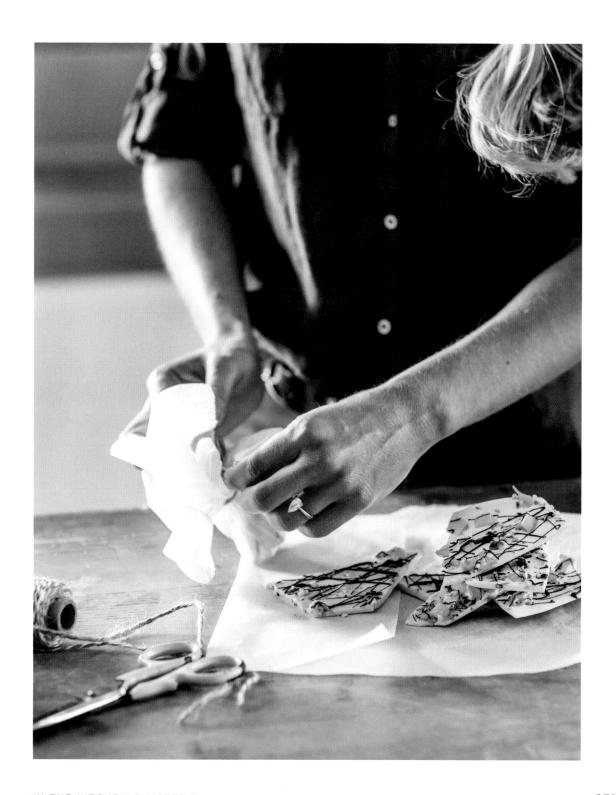

Live berry and coconut jelly

I've never met a jelly I didn't like, but this takes things to the next level. It's also won the heart of my two-year-old nephew = proud Aunty moment!

Base:

COCONUT LAYER:
5 leaves of gelatine
240g live coconut yoghurt
2 tbsp honey, or
  sweetener of choice

BERRY LAYER:
5 leaves of gelatine
145g frozen berries or
  mango
2 tbsp honey, or
  sweetener of choice

Coconut layer:

1. Place the gelatine sheets in a bowl and cover with cold water for 5 minutes to allow the gelatine to soften, then drain off the water.

2. Add 120ml of warm water to the gelatine. Stir until the gelatine has dissolved (approx. 30 seconds) and allow to cool.

3. Combine the coconut yoghurt and honey into a pouring jug before slowly stirring in the gelatine. Mix until smooth.

4. Using a flavourless oil or cake-release spray, lightly grease a jelly mould (or 15cm-diameter cake tin).

5. Pour the coconut layer into the bottom of the mould, leaving room for the berry layer. Place in the fridge to set overnight (or for at least 4 hours) before preparing the berry layer.

Berry layer:

1. Repeat step 1 above.

2. Place the berries and 250ml of warm water into a small blender, and allow to defrost for a few minutes before blending for a few seconds to form a rough purée.

3. Place the purée and honey into a saucepan and simmer over a low heat for 5 minutes, stirring every minute or so. Remove from the heat.

4. Place a metal sieve on top of a jug and pour the purée through it. With the back of a spoon, push all the pulp through the sieve, leaving just the seeds.

5. Add the softened gelatine to the purée and stir until dissolved. Once cooled to room temperature, spoon on top of the set coconut layer. Pop back in the fridge for 6–8 hours to set.

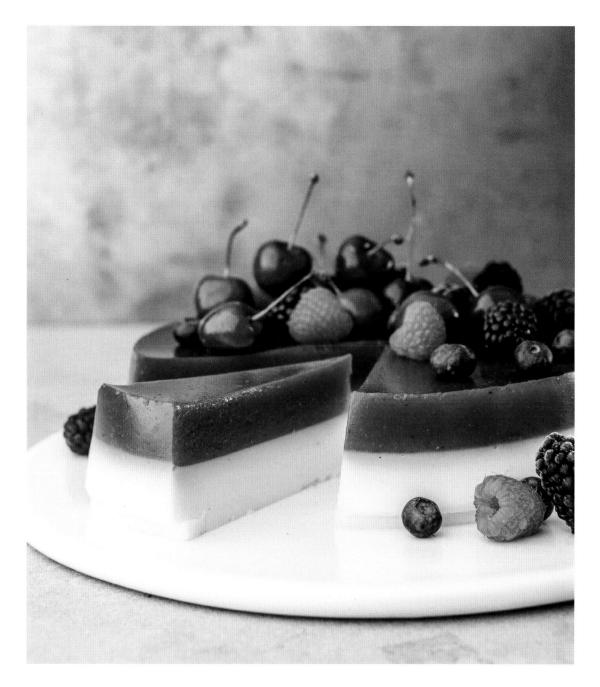

Options:

- Want a bit of extra texture? Stir 50g of desiccated coconut into the coconut layer before leaving to set.
- Don't throw out the seeds! They make a great addition to your breakfast granola.

Synbiotic ice-cream sticks

When convenience and taste align, you know you're on to a winner. No need for a fancy ice-cream machine, this combo draws on the creaminess of bananas and the richness of thick live yoghurt to deliver gut goodness on a stick.

Base:
1 ripe banana (the riper, the better; about 100g peeled weight)
2 Medjool dates, chopped and stirred into a paste with 1 tbsp of boiling water
240g live full-fat yoghurt of choice (dairy or coconut; see page 280)
1 tsp vanilla extract

Toppers
(choose one to mix in with the base):

1. NUTTY PISTACHIO:
(SERVES 6)
50g pistachios, shelled
10 baby spinach leaves (the chlorophyll in the leaves adds a touch of green to the ice cream)

2. RAW BANOFFEE:
(SERVES 8)
1 ripe banana (about 100g peeled weight)
120g coconut yoghurt
70g almond butter

Extra (optional):
dark chocolate
coconut flakes

1. Place all the base ingredients into a blender and blitz until smooth.

2. Choose your toppers and add into the base mix. Roughly blitz to your desired texture.

3. Spoon into setting moulds and place in the freezer for at least 4 hours.

4. Once set, warm the dark chocolate in the microwave for 40–60 seconds, if using, stirring vigorously every 15 seconds until melted. Lay the ice lollies on a lined baking tray, drizzle over the chocolate and sprinkle with coconut flakes, if using.

NB: If you struggle to get them out of the mould, dip the outside of the mould in warm water for a few seconds.

Options:
- Keep things simple and just mix in 50g of your fruit of choice to the base.
- Want to up the presentation stakes? Layer the moulds with different flavours, freezing before adding each one.

◆ *Can bacteria survive the freeze? You bet. According to research in the* Journal of Dairy Science, *they can't handle the heat, but they can handle the cold.*

◆ *Switching the cream for yoghurt will save you 86 per cent in greenhouse gas emissions.*

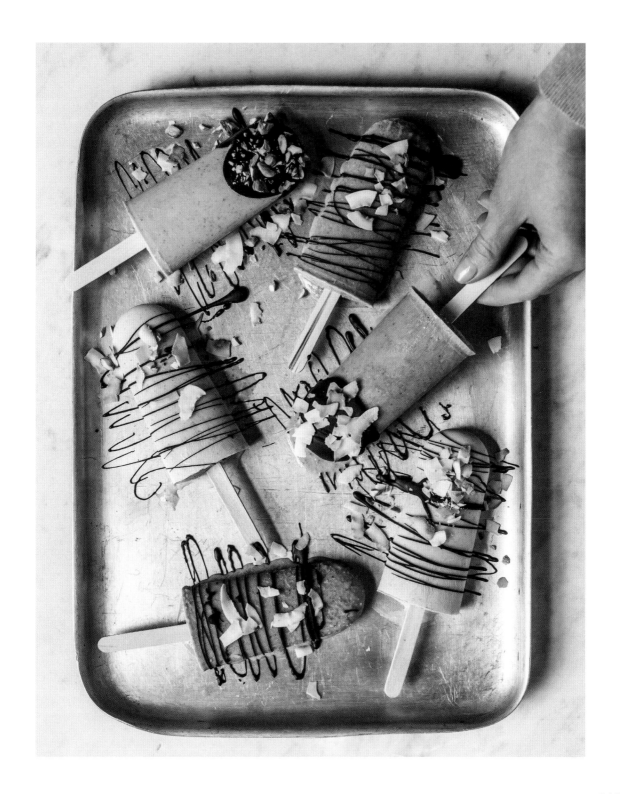

Welcome to fermenting!

What is fermentation?

Fermentation describes the process by which bacteria and yeast 'pre-digest' or transform food and drinks. In doing so, they produce a range of things (which scientists call 'by-products') such as vitamins, beneficial organic acids and other bioactive compounds, flavour compounds, gases and, in some cases, alcohol.

Unlike many fermenting advocates, who were born and raised on fermented goodness, fermenting isn't 'in my blood'. In fact, if you'd asked me only five years ago, I probably would have told you it was a bit too hippie dippie for me. But several years on, I've now realized I couldn't have been more wrong.

What began as a work-based experiment aimed at boosting my gut microbes rapidly turned into a deep-seated passion that's now embedded into my daily routine. During the experiment I noticed several things: I felt mentally and physically better than ever (anecdotal evidence alert: yes, that's the lowest-quality 'evidence' there is); my weekly grocery bill had reduced (hello, new shoes); and, above all, the thing that really got me hooked – the flavours. The microbes involved in fermentation possess the most extraordinary 'culinary' skills. You only have to think about the most flavoursome foods out there, such as aged cheeses, olives, chocolate, vanilla, coffee, wine and soy sauce, among others, none of which would be possible without microbes.

Before we get into the science of it, I want to tackle a few of the rumours about fermenting that could deter any budding fermenters out there ...

RUMOUR 1: **Fermenting is labour-intensive**

Fermenting reminds me of a slow cooker: it's surprisingly little effort – once you've prepared it, you just leave it, allow the microbes to do the heavy lifting and carry on with your activities. You later return to a dish that's transformed and ready to serve. It is true that some fermented foods can be a labour of love but, for those who are time poor, there are plenty of time-efficient options. Kefir, yoghurt and sourdough wraps all take about two minutes to prepare, you leave them overnight, and by morning they're ready to enjoy. Other ferments, such as kimchi and sauerkraut, take a little longer to prepare, but every few months I spend an afternoon making them in bulk.

RUMOUR 2: **Fermenting is dangerous**

Growing up in a generation where total sterilization was gospel and every household surface was soaked in anti-bacterial products, I was naturally a little intimidated by the perceived risk attached to fermenting. But it turns out the risk of food poisoning is far greater when you eat out at a restaurant. In fact, it's been suggested that regular consumption of traditional fermented foods may protect you from gut infections such as food poisoning – although I must admit most of the research is from animal studies.

You do need to keep your wits about you, use your senses (yes, the good old sniff test will tell you if something is rancid), and if in doubt ask for help (there is a very active Facebook fermenting community that is free to join).

RUMOUR 3: **Fermenting is not suitable for kids**

It's actually just the opposite and, in fact, I can't think of a better way to engage kids in science, food and healthy eating. Microbes, particularly yeast, do produce alcohol, but in most types of ferments the alcohol levels are below detection levels (i.e. considered alcohol-free), thanks to bacteria which convert the alcohol into beneficial organic acids.

> *Like dietary fibre, going from little to loads of fermented food within a few days can, in some people, trigger gut symptoms such as extra gas and bloating – think microbial party in a normally quiet neighbourhood. It's best to gradually increase the amount in your diet over several weeks. People with histamine sensitivity (see page 118) may need to limit their intake. And those with a weakened immune system or who are pregnant should discuss with a healthcare professional first.*

The process

Despite there being hundreds of different types of ferments, there are three main principles that underpin them all.

- MICROBES: No surprises here: in order to ferment, you need live microbes. There are two main types of ferments, determined by where the microbes come from. 'Wild ferments' use the microbes naturally found on plants and in the air, whereas 'culture-based ferments' involve adding a select group of microbes; think open house party (wild ferments, e.g. kimchi) versus invite-only parties (culture-based ferments, e.g. yoghurt).

- FOOD FOR THE MICROBES: The second most important ingredient is the food to keep the microbes alive. Without this, the microbes will become too weak to ferment. Like us, different microbes prefer different foods, which is why you need to be selective about the type of foods you feed different microbes. For example, the microbes used to make traditional yoghurt eat lactose (milk sugar), found in milk from animals. If you try adding these microbes to a lactose-free milk (e.g. plant-based milk), they starve and you are left with a watery mess instead of a thick, creamy yoghurt.

- SELECTIVE ENVIRONMENT: Just like some people prefer cold weather and others hot, different microbes prefer different types of environment. Ensuring the environment is matched to the microbes you're trying to grow will make sure you cultivate the right ones. For example, when fermenting vegetables, you need to create a salty, oxygen-free environment to support the growth of the lactic-acid bacteria while preventing the growth of fungi (surface mould) that can spoil your ferment. When it comes to the temperature, although most ferments do have an ideal temperature (detailed in each recipe), I've found most ferments can be pretty flexible. Also, within your home there are microclimates that you can make use of across seasons. For example, in winter I move my ferments closer to the airing cupboard. As a rule of thumb, microbes get rather sleepy and less active in cooler temperatures (which means ferments take longer) and more energized and active in warmer climates (ferments take less time).

Sprouting

One of the things I miss most about home is my mum's vegetable patch. There is something therapeutic about the process: planting the seeds, watching out for the first sprout, the daily watering and, finally, harvesting, preparing and eating the vegetables. While I certainly don't have the space (or time) to re-create my mum's luscious garden, I've found much of this gratification with sprouting.

The thing about sprouting is that anybody can do it anywhere; you don't need any fancy equipment or a lot of time. Sprouts are a great source of fibre and micronutrients and contain an array of polyphenols and other beneficial bioactive compounds. Studies have also shown that some types of sprouts contain manifold more bioactive compounds with anti-cancer benefits (albeit in test-tube studies), compared to the fully grown plants. Like fermenting, sprouting also decreases some types of anti-nutrients, as well as activating enzymes, and therefore increases the availability of several nutrients, such as amino acids (protein building blocks), and minerals, such as iron, calcium, magnesium and zinc.

That's not to say we should be ditching the fully grown plants and replacing them with sprouts; I consider them more of an extra kick of nutrients, rather than the bulk of my diet. For those wondering if there are any studies in humans, there aren't many. One trial did find that 60 grams of lentil sprouts eaten daily over eight weeks improved cholesterol levels as well as blood-sugar control in overweight people with type 2 diabetes. Sounds impressive, right? But annoyingly, because they didn't compare this to unsprouted lentils, it's impossible to know whether it was the act of sprouting or just the lentils themselves.

REST ASSURED: *It's not just about the health benefits – their nutty flavour and crunchy texture also make them a crowd-pleaser. Toss them into a salad, stir-fry, curry, burger or an omelette. While just about any bean, grain, vegetable, nut and seed can be sprouted, some are easier (and safer) than others. If you're new to sprouting, I recommend starting with an easy win – alfalfa seeds (page 278).*

Raw-slaw

Move over coleslaw, there's a new slaw in town – meet raw-slaw (aka sauerkraut): it's where the flavours (and microbes) are at. I put this on top of my burgers and as a side to all BBQ dishes. The process is simple – slice, salt, squash, submerge … sit.

Base:

300g Chinese cabbage, or cabbage of choice (I like to combine red and white varieties)

4g sea salt (or any non-iodized salt free of anti-caking agents)

1 tsp miso paste

1 spring onion, roughly chopped

1 tsp ginger, grated

Equipment:

500ml airtight jar, sterilized

Glass weight or mini glass jar to keep the ferment submerged

1. Rinse each of the cabbage leaves under running water (to get rid of any residual soil) before chopping to your desired thickness.

2. Put the sliced cabbage into a large bowl, then add the salt. Having cleaned your hands, firmly massage the salt into the cabbage until the cabbage is bruised – this process helps the microbes get into the cabbage cell walls, where they will do their thing.

3. Drain off a tablespoon of the cabbage juice that you have massaged out into a small mug and stir in the miso paste. Pour the miso over the bruised cabbage, along with the spring onion and ginger, and continue massaging the cabbage.

4. Transfer the mixture into a jar and, using your fist, punch down the slaw, pushing out all the air bubbles so there is a layer of juice separating the slaw and the air above it.

5. To keep the slaw submerged, place a glass weight or mini jar on top of the slaw.

6. Screw the lid on to the jar and leave at room temperature (ideally, 18–22°C), out of direct sunlight. Each day, check on your ferment and release any gas that has built up by twisting the lid a little to let it escape.

7. After 7 days (more in colder climates, less in warmer climates), your slaw is ready to taste. If you're new to fermenting, that might be sufficient time; if you prefer a stronger acidic flavour, continue to ferment for up to 4 weeks, testing weekly. Once it has reached your preferred flavour, pop it into the fridge for a few days to allow the flavour to rest before tucking in (this puts the microbes to sleep, limiting further fermentation).

Role of salt

I am normally all for limiting salt, but when it comes to fermented vegetables salt has several important functions. **1.** It creates a selective environment which supports the beneficial lactic acid bacteria, which, unlike many microbes, are rather salt-tolerant; **2.** Through a process known as osmosis, salt helps to draw the juices out of the vegetables, providing the liquid needed to submerge the vegetables; **3.** It preserves the crisp crunch of cabbage that would otherwise turn mushy.

The 'sweet' salt spot is around 1.5–2 per cent by weight of vegetables. It's best to weigh your salt because, depending on the grain size, volumes can yield very different weights. If you're limiting your salt, ferments can still work with lower levels of salt, but they won't last as long. Non-iodized salt free of anti-caking agents is best.

For those worried about the effect of added salt on blood pressure, there is some evidence to suggest it's probably not as detrimental as salt from processed foods. This is likely owing to the potassium-rich vegetables, which are known to lower blood pressure and therefore may offset the impact of the salt. One study reported that a daily intake of 210 grams of kimchi for seven days did not impact blood pressure, although this was in people with a healthy blood pressure. Nonetheless, if you do have high blood pressure or are concerned, it's a good idea to discuss with your health-care professional. You might also like to do a mini trial on yourself, testing the impact of regularly consuming fermented vegetables on your blood pressure over a few weeks.

Tap Water

Chlorine is another microbe inhibitor, which is why it's added to drinking water in the first place. Rather than buying filtered or spring water, you can de-chlorinate your tap water by boiling it with the lid open so that the chlorine can escape. Allow it to cool before using (hot water will kill the microbes).

Mould

If you notice any surface mould growing, it may be because you didn't completely submerge your vegetables. While some people say you can just scrape it off and continue fermenting, I like to play it safe, which means ditching and starting again.

Kimchi

An iconic condiment in Korean culture, this ancient flavour bomb is said to be one of the secrets behind the Koreans' long and healthy lives. In fact, a study published in the *Lancet* (top journal) has forecasted that South Korean women will be the first in the world to have an average life expectancy above ninety years by 2030.

Base:
200g Chinese cabbage, or cabbage of choice
25g sea salt (don't worry: you won't be eating this!)

Toppers:
50g carrot, grated (approx. 1 carrot)
1 spring onion, diced
50g daikon radish, chopped into matchsticks
1 clove of garlic, finely sliced
1 tsp ginger, grated
1 tsp gochugaru powder (available online or at Asian grocers. In its place use ½ tsp chilli powder and ½ tsp paprika)
1 tbsp tamari (or soy sauce)

Equipment:
500ml glass jar, with lid

1. Rinse the cabbage leaves under running water (to get rid of any residual soil) before chopping to the desired thickness.

2. Put the cabbage and salt in a bowl. Firmly massage the salt into the cabbage.

3. Pour 500ml of water, filtered or de-chlorinated, over the cabbage and submerge it by sitting a plate on top. Let it soak for 2 hours.

4. Drain the soaked cabbage, and rinse three times to get rid of the excess salt. Squeeze out any excess water in the cabbage and place back in a bowl.

5. Add all the topper ingredients and mix well, before transferring the mixture into a 500ml jar and, using your fist, punching down so there's a layer of juice separating the raw kimchi and the air above.

6. Place your glass weight or mini jar on top of the raw kimchi, making sure to submerge all the vegetables.

7. Screw the lid on and leave at room temperature (ideally, 18–22°C), out of direct sunlight. Each day, check on your kimchi and release any gas that has built up by untwisting the lid a little to let it out.

8. After 3 days (more in colder climates, less in warmer climates) your kimchi is ready for its first taste. If you're missing that acidic bite, leave for an extra day or two.

9. Once it's reached your preferred flavour, pop it in the fridge with the lid sealed tight to trap in the gas, creating the fizziness of traditional kimchi. Leave it for 2 weeks to allow the flavours to develop. Enjoy with eggs (my favourite), salads or feta on crackers – the options are endless.

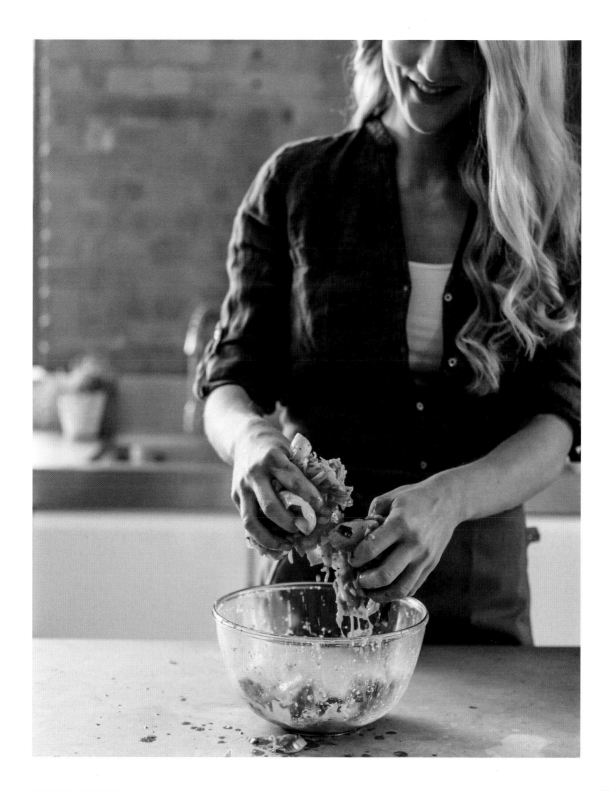

Sourdough starter

When I first started making sourdough I was gifted a starter from my local artisan bakery. As I became more confident with the process, I wanted to challenge myself to see whether I could make a starter from scratch. It does take more time and requires a bit more fermenting experience, but it's something you only need to do once – if you look after it, it can keep for ever.

Each day for 7 days:
¼ a cup of strong white flour

Equipment:
400ml glass jar
muslin/ cheesecloth (to cover)
rubber band

1. Day 1: In the glass jar, stir together the flour and a quarter of a cup of hand-warm water (add the water to the flour to prevent clumping). Cover with the muslin cloth and secure with a rubber band. Leave overnight at room temperature (ideally, 20–24°C).

2. Day 2: In the morning, stir and cover again. That evening, stir before discarding all but 1 tablespoon of your floury mix, known as the 'starter'. To your starter, add fresh flour and water, repeating step 1.

◆ *Why throw out most of your starter? I am anti-food-waste, but this step is important when making a starter. This is because overwhelming the starter each day with more fresh food than there is starter lowers the acidity and gives the yeast a competitive advantage.*

3. Days 3–7: repeat step 2.

4. Day 8: In the morning, stir. Your starter should appear fluffy, with a network of bubbles throughout and have a slightly sour and yeasty smell. This means it's ready to be used in your sourdough recipes. If there are only a few bubbles, continue feeding your starter for a few more days until it becomes more active.

STORAGE TIPS:
Store your starter in the fridge, sealed with an airtight lid. As you use your starter, replace with equal parts flour and water to ensure you maintain it – you don't want to have to start again from scratch. At a minimum, feed your starter once a week with 1 tablespoon flour and 1 tablespoon water. Mix well and leave on the kitchen counter, covered with the muslin cloth, for 1–2 hours before returning to the fridge with the lid secured.

Sourdough wrap

I love sourdough bread, although the hours of leavening and dough stretching mean I rarely get time to make it. Instead of settling for the shop-bought stuff, I decided to experiment with fermented wraps. A few attempts later, a time-efficient sourdough victory was mine! It's now become my go-to sourdough fix.

Base:
100g wholemeal flour
1 teaspoon sourdough
  starter (see opposite)

Topper:
a pinch of salt

1. In a glass or ceramic bowl, whisk the flour, 150ml of water and the sourdough starter together. Cover with a clean cloth secured with a rubber band and leave at room temperature (ideally, 20–24°C), out of direct sunlight, for 6–8 hours (plus or minus a few hours, depending on the temperature), or until the batter becomes fluffy with a network of bubbles throughout. If you prefer a sourer wrap, leave for longer. When ready for cooking, stir in the salt.

2. Warm a little oil over medium heat in a non-stick frying pan. Add half a cup (120ml) of the batter to the pan and swirl around the pan for an even wrap.

3. Cook for approximately 1 minute, until there are bubbles in the wrap and you can lift it to flip easily.

4. Cook on the other side for a minute or until slightly brown. Wrap in a clean tea towel to keep in the moisture until ready to serve. Best eaten warm.

◆ *What's the deal with sourdough and fermented bread? The delicious taste and chewiness aside, sourdough fermentation has been shown to lower the blood-sugar response to bread and also to increase the bioavailability of nutrients (meaning that more nutrients are freed up for absorption). Better still, the microbes found in a sourdough starter have been shown to produce bioactive compounds with impressive antioxidant activity. Winning on all fronts.*

Dairy Kefir

Kefir, a cousin to yoghurt, has the same creaminess but provides a more diverse array of microbes. It also offers a refreshingly crisp bite, thanks to the organic acids which are produced by the millions of microbes that live together in the kefir grains in happy synergy. Like wine, kefir is more of an acquired taste, so don't be surprised if it takes a few goes before you're hooked.

Base:
400ml full-fat milk (the milk sugar, lactose, is the microbe's food, and the milk fat helps to protect the microbes during the transit through the acidic environment in the stomach)
1 tbsp kefir grains

Toppers (optional: second ferment):
½ a cup of extra-ripe berries or fruit of choice

Equipment:
sieve
funnel
wooden spoon
750ml glass jar with lid, sterilized
750ml glass bottle or jar for finished kefir

1. Pour the milk into a glass jar with the kefir grains. Stir and seal the lid (if you like a fizzy kefir) or loosely cover with the lid (if you prefer a flatter kefir). Kefir is impartial to oxygen. Leave at room temperature (ideally, 20–25°C) for 8 hours, out of direct sunlight. Periodically, shake the jar to circulate the grains.

2. Stir the kefir and taste (the milk, not the grains). If the milk is still a little watery, leave for a further 4–8 hours. Again, periodically shake the jar to circulate the grains. If you prefer a more sour-tasting milk or live in a cooler climate, you may wish to leave your ferment for up to 48 hours, but remember, if you've tightened the lid, be sure to release the gas by lifting the lid every 8 hours or so.

3. Once it's reached your desired taste and consistency, pour the kefir and grains through a sieve. Transfer the kefir milk to an airtight glass bottle and either store in the fridge ready for use or begin the optional second ferment. Depending on how often you drink the kefir, you can repeat the process by adding the strained grains into a fresh jar of milk, or store the grains (see storage tips on page 277).

4. *Optional second ferment:* Add the berries to the bottle of kefir milk. Stir and seal the lid (if you like a fizzy kefir) or loosely cover with the lid (if you prefer a flatter kefir). (This time around, the microbes feast on the fruit sugar, fructose.) How long you let your kefir ferment is up to you. Taste your kefir at least every 8 hours to get a feel for how the flavour changes over time (and, importantly, to let the built-up gas out). The second ferment can take anywhere from 8 to 48 hours, depending on the fermenting conditions.

5. Once you are happy with the taste, chill in the fridge, then serve.

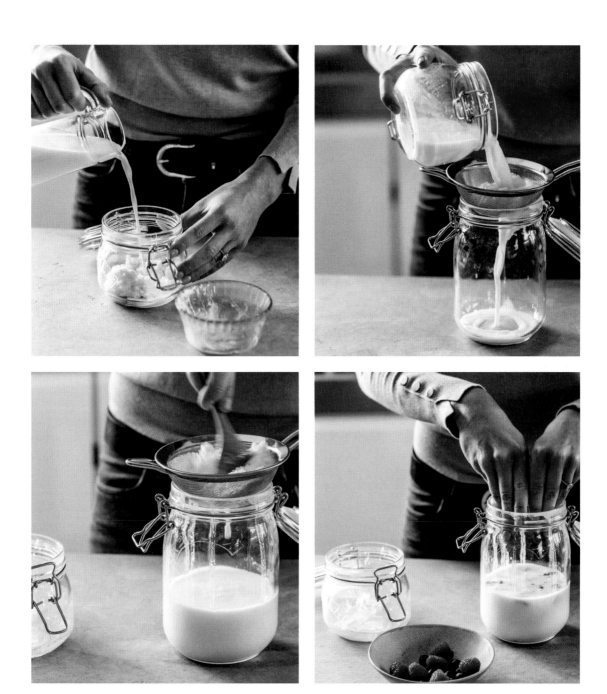

◆ *Fermentation produces a range of organic acids which give the kefir a pleasantly sour smell – this is completely normal. For those new to fermenting and a little hesitant, your senses will be quick to tell you if something's gone bad – trust me. If you need a reminder of the difference, go and smell some milk that has gone off.*

Water kefir

For those after a dairy-free drink, water kefir has you covered. Although not directly related to dairy kefir, the grains look similar although more translucent, as in the picture opposite. The dairy kefir survives on lactose (milk sugar), whereas the water kefir thrives on sucrose (table/cane sugar).

Base:
2 tsp fresh lemon juice
2 tbsp sugar (white, brown, cane and rapadura sugar all work and create slightly different flavours)
2 tbsp water kefir grains
1 dried fig (free of sulphur-containing additives or oils. The fig adds a touch of nutrition for extra healthy microbes. Best to add in every third batch to avoid overfeeding)

Toppers (second ferment):
25g ripe berries or fruit of choice, chopped

Equipment:
sieve
funnel
wooden spoon
750ml jug
750ml glass jar with lid, sterilized
750ml air-tight glass bottle for finished kefir

1. Put 500ml of filtered warm water and lemon juice into a glass jar, add the sugar and dissolve. Once the water has cooled, add in the kefir grains and fig, then loosely cover with the lid. Leave at room temperature (ideally, 20–25°C) for 8–12 hours, out of direct sunlight. Periodically, shake the jar to circulate the grains.

2. Stir the kefir and taste (the water, not the grains). If the water is still completely flat and sweet, leave for a further 4–8 hours. Warning: water kefir grains are much more active then milk kefir so, if you do tighten the lid, be sure to release the pressure by loosening it every 4–8 hours, depending on your climate.

3. Once you can taste a slight fizz, pour the kefir and grains through a sieve, catching the kefir water in a jug. Transfer the kefir water to an airtight glass bottle (discard the fig). Depending on your kefir demand, you can repeat the process by adding the strained kefir grains into a fresh jar of sugar water, or store the grains (see storage tips opposite).

4. *Second ferment:* Add the fruit to the bottle of kefir water. Seal the lid to trap in the carbon dioxide, which gives that refreshing fizz. Periodically, shake the jar to circulate the grains. How long you let your kefir ferment is up to you. Taste your kefir at least every 4–8 hours to get a feel for how the flavour changes over time. If you forget to let the gas out every 4–8 hours, before doing so, place it in the fridge to cool down and open it away from your face outside – just to be on the safe side (like you would a champagne bottle – water kefir really can give off a big pop!) The second ferment can take anywhere from 4 to 24 hours, depending on the fermenting conditions and your taste preferences (the longer you leave it, the more acidic the bite).

5. Once you are happy with the taste, chill in the fridge, then serve.

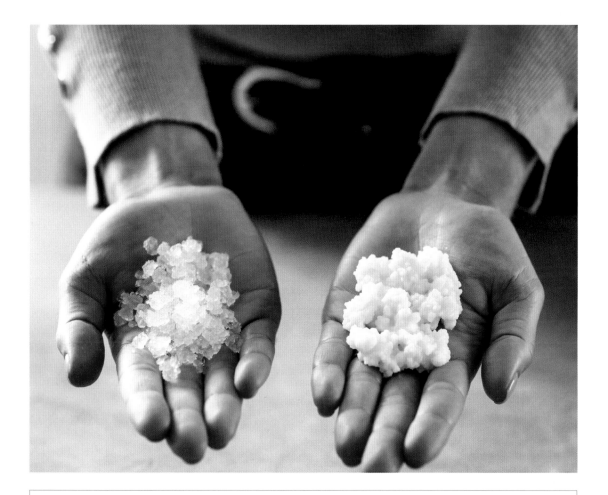

STORAGE TIPS:

- *Frequent consumer (at least 400ml a week): This is me: when my first batch of kefir is ready, I sieve out my grains and add them to a fresh jug of milk/sugary water, repeating step 1 and 2. Once it has reached a few hours shy of my desired taste, I pop the whole jar in the fridge, where I keep it until I've gone through my first batch of kefir. While it's in the fridge the fermentation continues, but at a much slower rate (dairy kefir keeps in the fridge for up to a week, water kefir two weeks). I then remove it from the fridge and follow step 3.*
- *Infrequent consumer (or when going on holiday): You have a few options. 1. Give to a friend to 'kefir-sit': add the grains to milk/sugar and store in the fridge with the lid sealed tight. Once a fortnight, your sitter will need to change the milk/sugary water. 2. Freeze: first pat the kefir grains dry, then place in an airtight container/zip-lock bag. When you return, place the frozen grains in milk/sugary water to defrost and start at step 1. It will take a few batches before your kefir is back to its bubbly self.*

◆ *Your kefir grains will double in size every few weeks. As the proportion of grains to milk/sweet water increases, it will ferment faster and faster. It's best to keep the grain:milk/water ratio at around 5 per cent and 8 per cent, respectively, to prevent over-fermenting. Why not gift your excess grains to friends and family?*

Sprouting seeds and legumes

This is a staple in my gut-goodness bowls. Don't feel you should be limiting them to one dish, though; the nutty flavours and crispy crunch make for the perfect high-protein topper in any meal.

Base:
¼ a cup of alfalfa sprouting seeds or dried peas or chickpeas (to be extra safe, it's best to buy seeds and legumes specifically for home sprouting; they're available from most garden centres)

Equipment:
wide-mouthed 600ml glass jar, sterilized muslin/cheesecloth (to cover)
rubber band
sieve

1. **Day 1:** Using a sieve, rinse the seeds/legumes well. Place them in a jar and cover with three-quarters of a cup of water (the seeds/legumes will increase a lot in size, so resist the temptation to add extra seeds into the jar). Cover the jar with cloth and secure with a rubber band. Leave to soak overnight at room temperature (ideally, 18–24°C).

2. **Day 2:** In the morning, using a sieve, drain off the water, rinse and drain again. Cover again with the cloth. Invert the jar and rest it at an angle, using the side of a bowl to hold the bottom of the jar up. This will allow the air to circulate and excess water to drain off. In the evening, repeat the rinsing and draining procedure – this is important to prevent mould from growing on your sprouts (in warm climates, you may need to repeat the rinsing and draining process up to four times a day).

3. **Days 3–8:** Repeat step 2, until 90 per cent of the seed jackets have fallen off (in the case of alfalfa) or once the tails are as long as the legume itself.

4. **Day 9:** Rinse and drain one last time before: (alfalfa) patting dry, placing in an airtight sterilized jar and storing in the fridge ready to eat; or (legumes) adding to a saucepan of water and bringing to the boil. Reduce the heat and boil gently for 45 minutes (for a more firm legume to add to salads), or 60 minutes (for a softer legume perfect for hummus; see recipe on page 240). Let cool, pat dry and store in an airtight sterilized jar in the fridge, ready to use.

STORAGE TIPS:
- *Alfalfa will last in the fridge for 1–2 weeks.*
- *For the legumes, cook first, and they will keep in the fridge for around 4 days.*

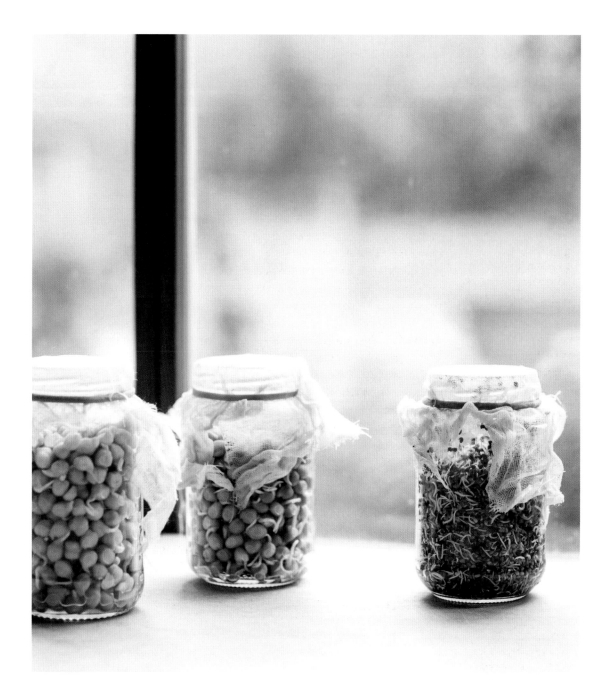

◆ *Broccoli sprouts are one of the best sources of a phytochemical called glucosinolate. Glucosinolates are converted (with the helping hand of your GM) into the almighty antioxidant sulforaphane. This phytochemical is linked with a decreased risk of cancer and heart disease.*

Live yoghurt

Not only does yoghurt make a great snack on its own, its creamy consistency has earned it a place in many of my recipes, including sauces, dips and baking. The benefits of yoghurt extend beyond the live microbes. Alongside the lactic acid, it also provides 25 per cent of most people's daily calcium needs.

Base:
2 tbsp live plain yoghurt (check the label for a yoghurt which contains 'live cultures' or 'probiotics')
600ml full-cream milk (full-cream milk makes a thicker, creamier yoghurt)

Topper: blueberry chia jam (optional)
140g blueberries (or berry of choice)
1 Medjool date, chopped
1 tbsp chia seeds

Equipment:
ovenproof jar, sterilized thermometer

STORAGE TIP:
• Yoghurt: keeps in the fridge for up to a week.
• Chia jam: keeps in the fridge for up to 2 weeks.

The yoghurt:

1. Place the milk in a saucepan on a low–medium heat and gently simmer until it reaches around 45°C.

2. Put the yoghurt (the source of microbes) into an ovenproof jar and slowly stir in the warmed milk so that the yoghurt is evenly dispersed.

3. Now to create the warm environment – their preferred temperature is around 40–45°C – that makes the yoghurt microbes flourish. There are several methods (including yoghurt makers, which I now use), but the oven works just fine. Heat the oven to 50°C fan, then turn it off. Turn on the oven light, then place the open jar in the oven. The light will keep the oven at a consistent temperature of around 40–45°C/105–115°F. Leave the jar in the oven for 8–12 hours. The longer the incubation period, the thicker and more tart the yoghurt.

4. Carefully remove the jar of yoghurt from the oven; allow it to cool on the kitchen counter before placing in the fridge to set.

Options:

• Add in 1 tbsp of milk powder in step 1 for an extra-thick yoghurt.

The blueberry chia jam:

1. Put the blueberries into a small saucepan, then add the chopped date and half a cup of water. Bring to a gentle simmer (don't boil). Using the back of a spatula, squish the blueberries and chopped dates, then simmer for 10 minutes.

2. Stir in the chia seeds and continue to simmer until the mixture starts to thicken (2–3 minutes). Take off the heat and let it cool.

3. Stir through a scoop of the jam with each serving of yoghurt.

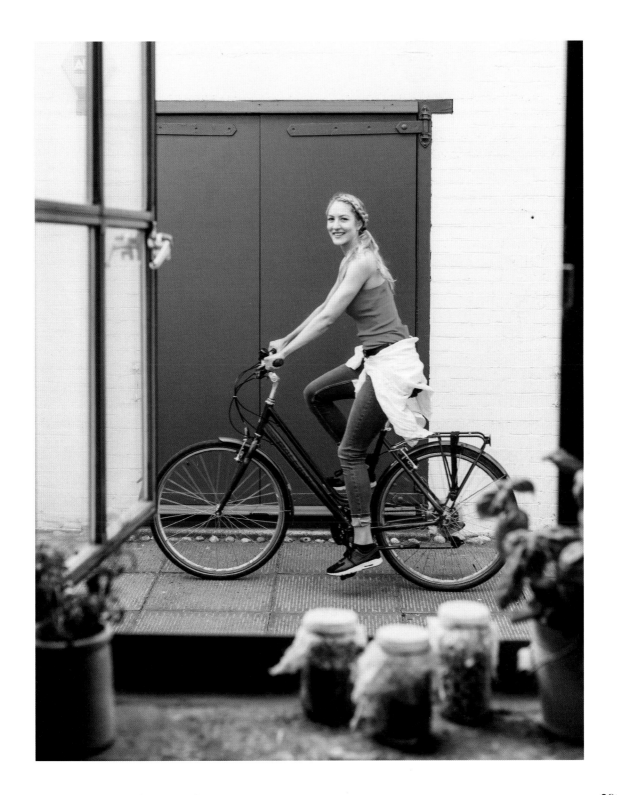

Conclusion:

Your Gut Health Action Plan

This is where change begins and results are achieved. This section is all about personalizing this book to reflect your very own unique gut-health journey and goals; no two people will be the same. We will bring together all the knowledge you have taken the time to learn in going through this book, and the assessments you have completed, to help prioritize and plan your next steps.

Consider this space your activity pad – this is where you can record the results from each of the assessments, along with any of the specific strategies that you feel are relevant and feasible for you. You can also jot down any extra notes to help consolidate different concepts presented in the book. There is no wrong or right way of doing this: you can complete as many or as few of the sections, and whether you start today or in a few months, again, it's completely your call.

Making time

If you find yourself delaying things because you feel you just don't have the time, I want you to stop for a moment and imagine life with fewer sick days and more productive days, without those gut issues, or even just feeling that little bit happier and more focused. Think of the time you would save, time you could reinvest into your family, friends, hobbies, work, or just you. Even if you start by spending just a few minutes each day implementing one of your strategies, isn't it worth a try?

Record your results from each assessment at www.TheGutHealthDoctor.com as you go through the book to help keep track of how things are progressing.

STEP 1:
Listening to your gut feelings
(page 21)

Taking the time to pinpoint any specific gut symptoms that are bothering you is an important first step to bringing about change. The type, location, frequency and severity of symptoms can help you select the right strategies to beat your symptoms for good.

DATE:..

GUT SYMPTOM SCORE:....................................

KEY SYMPTOMS:..

....

DO YOU HAVE ANY ALARM FEATURES?

....

STRATEGIES:..

....

....

....

REVIEW DATE:..

STEP 2:
Checking in with your poop
(page 21)

Okay, so it's not something we need to start discussing over dinner, but your poop is an invaluable resource when it comes to assessing your gut health. Inspecting every 'delivery' is certainly not required; instead, just keep an eye on what your average poop looks like.

DATE:..

FREQUENCY:...

TIME OF DAY:...

CONSISTENCY:...

COLOUR:...

AVERAGE DAILY POOP SIZE:............................

DO YOU HAVE ANY ALARM FEATURES?

....

STRATEGIES:..

....

....

REVIEW DATE:..

STEP 3:
How diverse is your GM? (page 29)

Our diet offers unique insight into our GM diversity. Because, after all, our microbes are completely reliant on what we feed them. Rest assured, we don't need to sacrifice taste and flavour, but just sparing a thought for our microbes at each meal can go a long way to improving not just their but our health and happiness, too.

DATE:...

FIBRE SCORE:..

DIET-DERIVED GM SCORE:..................................

STRATEGIES (don't forget those laid out in your plant-based diversity planner on page 76):

....

....

....

....

....

....

REVIEW DATE:..

STEP 4:
How happy are you? (page 33)

There is no escaping the link between our gut and our brain. And now, with trials demonstrating the impact of a 'gut-boosting' diet on mental health, there's a strong case for checking in with your happiness levels before and after implementing the strategies within this book.

DATE:...

SCORE:..

STRATEGIES:..

....

....

REVIEW DATE:..

STEP 5:
Gut–brain assessment (page 81)

For those who experience a collection of gut symptoms, it can be helpful to assess whether the gut–brain axis is involved in perpetuating them. Determining this will inform the most effective pathway needed to manage your symptoms.

DATE:...

SCORE:..

STRATEGIES:..

....

REVIEW DATE:..

STEP 6:
Are food intolerances to blame? (page 110)

Determining whether a food is the cause of your symptoms can be incredibly confusing. Instead, taking a systematic, evidence-based approach using the 3R Method can help cut through the misperceptions and fear attached to certain foods. This process will help to re-establish your relationship with food by getting to the bottom of suspected food intolerances, in turn empowering you to enjoy more foods with confidence.

DATE:..

RESULT OF STEP 1: RECORD:.........................

....

RESULT OF STEP 2: RESTRICT:.......................

....

....

....

RESULT OF STEP 3: REINTRODUCE:.................

....

....

....

PLAN:...

....

....

REVIEW DATE:......................................

STEP 7:
Is it IBS or another functional gut disorder? (page 139)

I'm not generally one for labels, but getting the right diagnosis is key to getting your symptoms under control. This is because it eliminates a lot of the trial and error, allowing you to choose more targeted strategies based on trials in people with the same diagnosis.

DATE:..

DO YOU NEED TO SEE YOUR GP?
If so, record date of appointment:

....

HAVE YOU BEEN TESTED FOR COELIAC DISEASE AND OTHER OVERLAPPED DISEASES? Record date and test results:

....

....

DO YOU FULFIL IBS CRITERIA?.....................

IBS SUBTYPE:.......................................

DO YOU HAVE ANOTHER FUNCTIONAL GUT DISORDER?..

STRATEGIES:.......................................

....

....

RESULT OF STAGE 1: RESTRICTION...

....

RESULT OF STAGE 2: REINTRODUCTION...

....

RESULT OF STAGE 3: PERSONALIZATION..

....

STEP 8:
Let's talk about sleep
(page 164)

Although it may sound like a no-brainer, too few of us are getting enough good-quality sleep. As we explored, improving your sleep can have far-reaching benefits, extending to diet, immunity, mood and focus. With that in mind, it's certainly worth considering your sleeping habits and testing out some of the sleep-hygiene strategies.

DATE:...

SCORE:...

STRATEGIES:..

....

....

....

REVIEW DATE:...

STEP 9:
How good is your immunity?
(page 20)

Are you constantly getting sick? It could be a tell-tale sign that you need to check in with your GM – how are you treating it? Yes, when it comes to your immunity, there are factors outside your control. But there are also a number of factors within your control: diet, sleep, stress and exercise all play an important part.

DATE:...

SCORE:...

STRATEGIES:..

....

....

....

REVIEW DATE:...

STEP 10:
Is stress getting the better of you? (page 167)

We've all experienced stress, and that's normal. But when it becomes a regular occurrence it can seriously impact your health and happiness. No one should have to live with the consequences of stress overload but, unfortunately, many of us do. Is stress affecting you?

DATE:..

SCORE:...

STRATEGIES:..

....

....

....

REVIEW DATE:...

STEP 11:
How active are you? (page 180)

You may always be rushing around and feel physically exhausted, but have you ever stopped and considered how your fitness levels stack up against recommendations? Sometimes it just takes a quick check for us to realize that we've got caught up in the daily grind, sporting a racing mind and an inactive body.

DATE:..

SCORE:...

STRATEGIES:..

....

REVIEW DATE:...

WHAT ABOUT YOUR BOWEL FITNESS AND TECHNIQUE? (pages 182–83)

....

ARE YOU A GOOD POOPER?............................

HOW STRONG IS YOUR PELVIC FLOOR?

....

....

STRATEGIES:..

....

REVIEW DATE:...

Forming new habits

Forming healthy habits isn't always easy. We often start with the best intentions but, within a few weeks or so, when the motivation starts to fade and the demands of life take over, we can find ourselves back at square one. To help combat this common pattern that can affect us all, I've listed my top habit-forming tips, which have been tried and tested by my patients.

- Form a trigger by attaching the activity to another habit, e.g. brushing your teeth.

- Set a daily reminder on your phone until the action becomes automatic.

- If you're into lists, start a daily tick-sheet.

- Keep the time and place consistent.

- Find a friend who may also benefit; you can then keep each other motivated.

- Leave a Post-it note on your bedroom mirror reminding you why you started.

- Record any good feelings or experiences related to the activity in a notepad.

- Celebrating any success, no matter how small, can really help reinforce your commitment.

- Don't be too hard on yourself if you miss a day or two; look forward to getting back to it tomorrow.

- Be realistic from the start: don't try to implement too many changes at once. If the activity calls for fifteen minutes a day but you only have ten minutes, just start with that. If it means you get started today, you'll still be one step ahead.

- If your motivation is running on empty, try bringing some emotion back into the activity by asking yourself two questions:

1

How will I feel if I continue versus if I stop?

2

What will my life look like in one year if I continue versus if I stop?

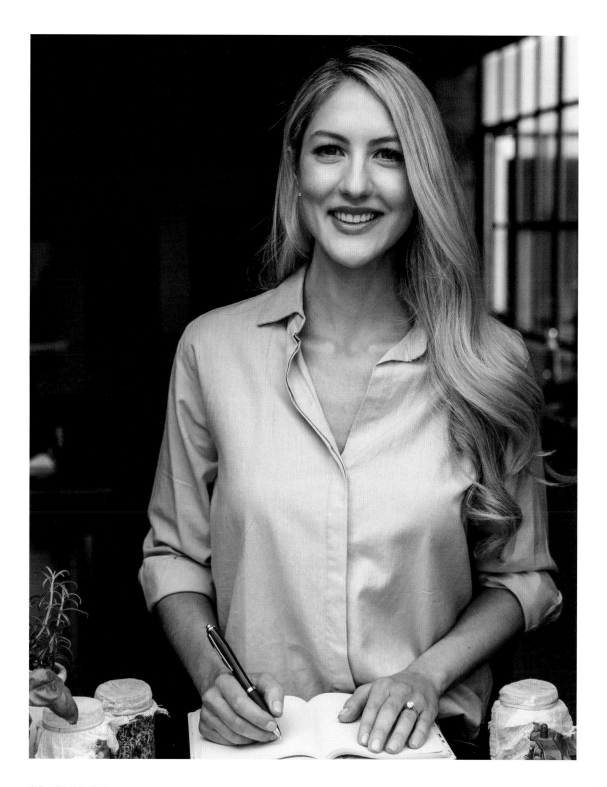

Final Word

So, there you have it – the foundation of your gut-health journey has been laid. It's really only the start but, undoubtedly, that's a victory in itself and something you should be unashamedly proud of. You have made a conscious decision to take charge of your health and happiness by beginning this journey of self-discovery and getting to know your GM and all its mind-blowing potential. With the intention of condensing and prioritizing all the things you've learned along the way, have a think about what your top three gut-health goals for the next six months might be.

Goal 1: NOTES:	
Goal 2: NOTES:	
Goal 3: NOTES:	

Over time, these may change, but setting yourself targets can keep you focused on what is most important to you.

I've personally seen this gut-health journey genuinely transform the lives of my patients and, importantly, it's not just my own experience talking, it's a powerful concept backed by a wealth of science, which continues to expand. Taking control of their gut health has helped people regain their confidence, improve their quality of life, revive their love of food, defy the odds and prevent family history of chronic diseases such as diabetes, as well as manage other conditions, including heart disease, and so much more. Gut health is truly revolutionizing our approach to health and wellness, and embracing this vast, untapped resource that lives within each and every one of us is a game-changer.

I hope this book continues to inspire you throughout your journey. No matter how slow or how small your steps, I promise you, it will be worth it. This area is not just my job, it's my passion, and for a long time I have wanted to put all the knowledge and real-world clinical experience I have gained, alongside the landmark research being done around the world, into one place that's easily accessible for all. I hope I've given you a framework with which you – anyone – can build your own unique gut-health journey and feel empowered to improve your health and happiness. I know you have so much potential to take this knowledge and continue on your journey, and I am confident you will see results. So, with that, I will leave it in your capable hands.

Index

A

acid reflux 102–5
air travel: and IBS 149
Al Khatib, Dr 164
alcohol: and IBS 143
Allen, Lucy 182
antibiotics 34, 55
  and diarrhoea 95
  and SIBO 156
artificial sweeteners *see*
  sweeteners

B

beetroot 200, 229
belly breath 173
bile acid diarrhoea (BAD) 157
bile acids 16
bloating 88–93
bowel massage 185
bowel-training exercises 180, 182–5
Bradshaw, Ellie 182
brahmari pranayama (humming-bee breath) 173
brain 10–11, 19, 32–3
breakfast recipes 194–207
breath 173
bridge pose 177
broccoli sprouts 279

C

caffeine sensitivity 119
  and IBS 143
calcium 69
carbohydrates 44–5
  see also fibre; FODMAPs
cat-cow 174
cauliflower 251
challenging judgemental thoughts 170
cheese 193
child's pose 174
chilli 143
chocolate 253, 258
circulation 30–31
Clostridioides difficile (C.diff) 27
cocoa 253, 258
cognitive behaviour therapy (CBT)
  166, 170
constipation 82–7
  and flatulence 99
corpse pose 177
crocodile twist 177
cumin 236

D

diaphragmatic breathing 173
diarrhoea 94–6
  and IBS 157

diet:
  and bloating 90, 92
  and constipation 84
  and diarrhoea 96
  diversity 29, 60, 68–77
  and exercise-associated gut
   discomfort 106
  and heartburn and acid reflux 104
  for IBS 141–8
  see also nutrition; recipes
dietary fibre see fibre
dieting 35
digestive system 14–17
dinner recipes 220–37
do-nothing exercise 168–9
down dog 175

E
eggs 193, 204
endometriosis 157
evacuation disorder 82
exercise 160–61, 180, 287
  bowel-training exercises 182–5
  and constipation 83, 85
  exercise-associated gut discomfort
   106–7
extra virgin olive oil (EVOO) 215, 225

F
faeces see poop
fasting 63
fats 44–5, 64
  and IBS 143

  omega-3 fats 65, 69
fermented foods 56–7, 71,
  264–7
  recipes 268–80
fibre 46–51
  and IBS 143, 154
flatulence 98–101
flaxseed 154
FODMAPs 118, 141, 145–53
  and bloating 92
  and exercise-associated gut
   discomfort 106
  recipe modifications 192
  spelt 247
food see diet; nutrition; recipes
food allergies 110–11
food intolerance: and bloating 92
food intolerances 110–13
  assessment 285
  caffeine 119
  diagnosing 121–33
  diet restriction 120
  fructose 118
  histamine intolerance 118
  lactose 114–15
  recipe modifications 192–3
  sulphite sensitivity 118
  what next? 134–5
  wheat and gluten 115–17
forward fold 175
fructans 116
fructose intolerance 118
fruit: and IBS 143, 151
functional gut disorders 88–9
  see also irritable bowel
  syndrome
fungi 26

G

garlic 235
gastro-oesophageal reflux disease (GORD) 102
ginger 221
gluten 117, 120
    intolerance 115–16, 123, 132–3
    and low-FODMAP diet 148
    recipe modifications 192
grains:
    fibre 47
    FODMAPs 151
greens 212
gut 6–9, 14–17
    common complaints 80–107
    and food intolerances 110–35
    gut-feelings assessment 21, 81, 283
    gut-health assessment 9, 285
    and IBS 138–57
    and immune system 20–21
    motility 18–19
    and nutrition 40–77
gut-associated lymphoid tissue (GALT) 20
gut–brain axis 10–11, 19, 32–3, 81
    and bloating 92
    and food intolerances 121
    gut–brain assessment 81, 284
    IBS 139
    stress 166–79
gut diary 123, 124–5, 144
gut-directed yoga flow 172–9
gut-health action plan 282–91
gut–kidney axis 10
gut microbiota (GM) 6, 14, 17, 26–9, 37
    and dieting 35
    diversity 29, 284
    and exercise 160–61, 180–85
    and health and well-being 30–31

and medication 28, 34
and sleep 35, 160–61, 162–5
and stress 160–61, 166–79
vulnerabilities 34–5

H

half-cobra 175
happiness 33, 284
happy baby 177
heartburn 102–5
herbs 71, 75
high-fructose corn syrup (HFCS) 118
histamine intolerance 118
humming-bee breath (brahmari pranayama) 173
hydration:
    and exercise-associated gut
        discomfort 106
    and fibre 50
    IBS 143
    and large intestine 17
    see also water
hygiene hypothesis 21

I

IgG tests 121
immune system 20–21, 30–31, 163, 286
inflammatory bowel disease (IBD): gut
    microbiota 26
intestine 16–17, 20
iodine 69
iron 69
irritable bowel syndrome (IBS) 116, 138
    and air travel 149

assessment 139, 285
cause 139
constipation 82
diagnosing 139
diet approach 141–53
and fasting 63
and fibre supplements 154
and FODMAPs 118, 145–53
and food intolerances 110, 112, 113, 135
and menstruation 157
and parasites 26
and peppermint oil 155
post-infectious IBS 94
and probiotics 54–5
and SIBO 156
and stress 166–7
support 157
ispaghula 154

K

kidneys 10

L

lactose intolerance 114–15, 123, 129, 130–31, 134
  and FODMAPs 148
  recipe modifications 192
large intestine 17
laxatives 86
leaky gut 20
legumes 71
lifestyle 34–5, 160–61
  and bloating 91
  and constipation 84–5

and diarrhoea 96–7
and heartburn and acid reflux 105
  see also exercise; sleep; stress
linseed 154
locust pose 176
lunch recipes 208–19

M

macronutrients 44–5
mass movement 19
meal planning 189–90
medication 28, 34
  see also antibiotics
menstruation 157
mental health 32–3
microbes 24–5
  in fermented foods 56, 57, 266
  see also gut microbiota; probiotics
microbiome 27
microbiota 27
micronutrients 44
migrating motor complex (MMC) 18
mindfulness exercise 178–9
minerals 44
mould: fermented foods 269
mouth 14
  microbiota 25
mushrooms 203

N

nervous system 30–31
non-coeliac gluten sensitivity 115–16
nutrition 40–43

additional nutrients 64–5
diet restriction 120, 128
dietary fibre 46–51
fasting 63
fermented foods 56–7
food additives 66
food form 62
gut-health eating 68–77
macronutrients 44–5
phytochemicals 58–9
plant-based-diet diversity 60, 68–77
prebiotics 52
probiotics 54–5
nutritional yeast 193
nuts 193

O

oats 199
oesophagus 15
heartburn and acid reflux 102–5
olive oil 205, 215, 225
omega-3 fats 65, 69
oral allergy syndrome (OAS) 111
oral microbiota 25

P

parasites 26
pelvic floor 183–4
peppermint oil 155
physical activity see exercise
phytochemicals 58–9, 209
pigeon pose 176
plant-based foods 62, 71

diet diversity 60, 73–4
month planner 76–7
nutrients 69
pollen-food syndrome (PFS) 111
polyphenols 44, 58–9
poop 17, 19
bowel-training exercises 182–3
checking in with your poop assessment 21
and fibre 46
and FODMAPs 146
gut-health assessment 283
and psyllium 154
see also constipation; diarrhoea
poop-pourri 87
prebiotics 9, 44, 52
probiotics 54–5
and skin microbiota 24–5
protein 44–5, 64
FODMAPs 151
psyllium 154

R

recipes 188
breakfast 194–207
dinner 220–37
fermented foods 268–80
lunch 208–19
meal planning 189–90
modifications for food intolerances 192–3
snacks 238–63
rectocele 82
relaxation techniques 166
do-nothing exercise 168–9
mindfulness exercise 178–9
resistant starch 212

S

sage twist 176
salt 67
  fermented foods 269
seaweed 219
selenium 69
short-chain fatty acids (SCFAs) 46
skin microbiota 24–5
sleep 18, 35, 160–61, 162–5, 286
slow-transit constipation 82
small intestinal bacterial
  overgrowth (SIBO) 18, 156
  and flatulence 99
small intestine 16
snacks:
  recipes 238–63
  on the run 191
spelt 247
spices 71, 75
sprouting 267, 278–9
stomach 15
stomach pain: IBS 155
stress 160–61, 166–7, 287
  challenging judgemental thoughts 170
  do-nothing exercise 168–9
  strategies 168–70
  yoga 171–9
sulphite sensitivity 118
sweet potato 233
sweeteners 66
  and IBS 143

T

3R Method 121, 122–33
toilet habits 83, 85

V

vegetables: FODMAPs 151
viruses 26
vitamin B12 69
vitamins 44

W

walnuts 252
water:
  and fermentation 269
  and IBS 143
  see also hydration
Western diet 40
wheat 117
  intolerance 115–16, 123, 132–3
wholegrains 47
Wilson, Kimberly 168
wind *see* flatulence

Y

yeast 193
yoga 166, 171–9

Z

zinc 69

toilet positions 182
toilet spray 87
traveller's diarrhoea 94

Index of Recipes

A

alfalfa: sprouting seeds and legumes 278
aubergines:
    aubergine cannelloni 228
    chargrilled miso aubergine 232
    meatless meatballs in rich
     tomato sauce 234
avocado and feta slider 196

B

bananas:
    banana, fig and courgette breakfast
     loaf 206
    power plant pancakes 199
    synbiotic ice-cream sticks 262
    thick protein shake 196
basil:
    raw lasagne 213
    sautéed Brussels sprouts and
     tenderstem broccoli 214
BBQ vegan wings 250
beans:
    butterbean curry 221
    coconut-crusted green dippers 248
    mini shakshuka egg pots 204
    power plant pancakes 199
    sea salt and rosemary legume
     crunch 246

    spicy baked beans 205
    spicy bean burgers 236
    see also chickpeas; lentils
beetroot:
    aubergine cannelloni with
     beetroot salsa 228
    DIY granola 201
berries:
    blueberry chia jam 280
    live berry and coconut jelly 260
    power plant pancakes 199
black bean brownies 253
blueberry chia jam 280
borlotti beans: spicy baked beans
  205
bowls: mix-and-match gut-
  goodness bowls 222–3
bread:
    sourdough starter 272
    sourdough wrap 273
broccoli: sautéed Brussels sprouts
  and tenderstem broccoli 214
broccoli sprouts: sprouting seeds
  and legumes 278
brownies: fudgy black bean
  brownies 253
Brussels sprouts and tenderstem
  broccoli 214
buckwheat and oat pizza 231

burgers: spicy bean burgers 236
butterbeans:
    butterbean curry 221
    mini shakshuka egg pots 204
butternut squash:
    butterbean curry 221
    Korean BBQ squash taco shells
      with kimchi 216

C

cabbage:
    kimchi 270
    raw-slaw 268
cannellini beans: power plant
    pancakes 199
cannelloni: aubergine cannelloni
    228
carrots:
    fermented overnight oats 195
    raw carrot cake balls 252
cashews:
    aubergine cannelloni with
      cashew cheese 228
    lemon curd in chia and cashew
      tartlets 257
    raw lasagne 213
cauliflower: sticky BBQ vegan wings
    250
cheese:
    avocado and feta slider 196
    chickpea crêpes with creamy
      feta and fungi 202
    pearl couscous in chicory boats
      212
cheesy vegan crackers 245
chia seeds:

blueberry chia jam 280
    lemon curd in chia and cashew
      tartlets 257
chickpeas:
    chickpea crêpes 202
    hummus 240
    pearl couscous in chicory boats 212
    spiced chickpea and sesame
      seed crackers 245
    sprouting seeds and legumes 278
    sweet potato and pulsing frittata 209
chicory: pearl couscous in chicory boats
    212
chocolate bark 258
cinnamon-spiced popcorn 254
cocoa:
    fermented overnight oats 195
    fudgy black bean brownies 253
coconut:
    coconut-crusted green dippers 248
    live berry and coconut jelly 260
corn: cinnamon-spiced popcorn 254
courgettes:
    banana, fig and courgette
      breakfast loaf 206
    fermented overnight oats 195
    raw lasagne 213
    sweet potato and pulsing frittata 209
couscous: pearl couscous in chicory
    boats 212
crackers:
    cheesy vegan crackers 245
    mix-and-match sliders 210
    seedy oatcakes 243
    spiced chickpea and sesame
      seed crackers 245
crisps: sesame and kale crisps 239
curry: butterbean curry 221

D

dates: raw carrot cake balls 252
dips 240
    harissa red pepper dip 242
    hummus 240
    pea and mint hummus 242
    zesty salsa dip 248

E

eggs:
    mini shakshuka egg pots 204
    power plant pancakes 199
    spicy baked beans 205
    sweet potato and pulsing frittata 209
    two-minute scram 196

F

feta cheese:
    avocado and feta slider 196
    chickpea crêpes with creamy
      feta and fungi 202
    pearl couscous in chicory boats 212
figs: banana, fig and courgette
    breakfast loaf 206
flaxseeds: cheesy vegan crackers 245
frittata: sweet potato and pulsing
    frittata 209

G

grains:
    mix-and-match gut-goodness
    bowls 222–3
    mix-and-match porridge 198
granola:
    DIY granola 201
    live breakfast parfait 196
green beans: coconut-crusted
    green dippers 248
greens:
    satay tofu skewers 226
    see also basil; kale; spinach

H

harissa red pepper dip 242
hazelnuts: harissa red pepper dip
    242
hummus 240
    pea and mint hummus 242

I

ice-cream sticks 262

J

jelly: live berry and coconut jelly 260

K

kale: sesame and kale crisps 239
kefir 274
    fermented overnight oats 195
    mix-and-match porridge 198
    thick protein shake 196

water kefir 276
kimchi 270
   Korean BBQ squash taco shells
    with kimchi 216
Korean BBQ squash taco shells
   with kimchi 216

L

lasagne 213
lemon curd in chia and cashew
   tartlets 257
lentils:
   lentil and mushroom fettuccine 237
   sweet potato and pulsing frittata 209

M

meatless meatballs in rich tomato sauce
   234
milk:
   kefir 274
   live yoghurt 280
mint: pea and mint hummus 242
miso: chargrilled miso aubergine 232
mix-and-match gut-goodness
   bowls 222–3
mix-and-match porridge 198
mix-and-match sliders 210
mozzarella: pearl couscous in
   chicory boats 212
mushrooms:
   chickpea crêpes with creamy
    feta and fungi 202
   lentil and mushroom fettuccine 237

N

nori: quinoa sushi rolls 219

O

oats:
   buckwheat and oat pizza 231
   DIY granola 201
   fermented overnight oats 195
   meatless meatballs in rich
    tomato sauce 234
   mix-and-match porridge 198
   power plant pancakes 199
   seedy oatcakes 243
olive pesto 228
onions:
   caramelized onions 236
   quinoa sushi rolls 219
overnight oats 195

P

pancakes:
   chickpea crêpes 202
   power plant pancakes 199
pasta 212
   creamy pistachio and spinach
    pesto pasta 225
   lentil and mushroom fettuccine 237
peanut butter:
   peanut and pear open sandwich 197
   satay tofu skewers 226
pearl couscous in chicory boats 212
pears: peanut and pear open
   sandwich 197

peas:
   pea and mint hummus 242
   sprouting seeds and legumes 278
peppers:
   harissa red pepper dip 242
   mini shakshuka egg pots 204
pesto:
   creamy pistachio and spinach
    pesto pasta 225
   olive pesto 228
   sautéed Brussels sprouts and
    tenderstem broccoli 214
   spinach and walnut pesto 213
pistachios:
   creamy pistachio and spinach
    pesto pasta 225
   synbiotic ice-cream sticks 262
pizza:
   buckwheat and oat pizza 231
   spelt and quinoa pizza 230
popcorn: cinnamon-spiced
   popcorn 254
porridge 198
prebiotic chocolate bark 258

Q

quinoa:
   quinoa sushi rolls 219
   spelt and quinoa pizza 230

R

raw-slaw 268
rice: sautéed Brussels sprouts and
   tenderstem broccoli 214
rosemary: sea salt and rosemary
   legume crunch 246

S

salsa: beetroot salsa 228
satay tofu skewers 226
sauerkraut 268
sea salt and rosemary legume crunch
   246
seedy oatcakes 243
sesame seeds:
   sesame and kale crisps 239
   spiced chickpea and sesame
    seed crackers 245
shakshuka egg pots 204
skewers: satay tofu skewers 226
slaw 268
sliders:
   avocado and feta slider 196
   mix-and-match sliders 210
sourdough starter 272
sourdough wrap 273
spelt:
   spelt and quinoa pizza 230
   spelt wraps 247
spinach:
   creamy pistachio and spinach pesto
    pasta 225
   raw lasagne 213
   synbiotic ice-cream sticks 262
sprouting seeds and legumes 278
sprouts *see* Brussels sprouts
squash *see* butternut squash
sticky BBQ vegan wings 250

strawberries: power plant
   pancakes 199
sushi: quinoa sushi rolls 219
sweet potatoes:
   chargrilled miso aubergine with
    sweet potato wedges 232
   power plant pancakes 199
   spicy bean burgers 236
   sweet potato and pulsing
    frittata 209
synbiotic ice-cream sticks 262

T

tacos: Korean BBQ squash taco
   shells with kimchi 216
tahini:
   hummus 240
   pea and mint hummus 242
   sesame and kale crisps 239
tahini dressing 232
teff grain: banana, fig and
   courgette breakfast loaf 206
tenderstem broccoli: sautéed
   Brussels sprouts and tenderstem
   broccoli 214
tofu:
   satay tofu skewers 226
   thick protein shake 196
tomatoes:
   buckwheat and oat pizza 231
   meatless meatballs in rich
    tomato sauce 234
   mini shakshuka egg pots 204
   pearl couscous in chicory boats
    212

raw lasagne 213
spelt and quinoa pizza 230
spicy baked beans 205

W

walnuts:
   raw carrot cake balls 252
   raw lasagne 213
water kefir 276
wraps:
   mix-and-match sliders 210
   sourdough wrap 273
   spelt wraps 247

Y

yoghurt 280
   coconut-crusted green dippers
    248
   live berry and coconut jelly 260
   live breakfast parfait 196
   mix-and-match porridge 198
   synbiotic ice-cream sticks 262

With thanks . . .

To my husband, it turns out you're not only a brilliant GP, but you have a real flare for editing. Thank you for coming on this journey with me and reading every single word (five times over). Mum, no words can describe how grateful I am for your endless support; without you there would be no book.

To my nutrition and dietetic colleagues who critically reviewed and challenged every page, you have made this book really something special: Dr Heidi Staudacher, Marianne Williams, Dr Katrina Campbell, Yvonne McKenzie, Dr Eirini Dimidi, Dr CK Yao, Dr Caroline Tuck, Dr Samantha Gill, Dr Ricardo Da Costa and Dr Ana Rodriguez-Mateos.

To the microbe experts, Dr Johan van Hylckama Vlieg, Dr Erin Shanahan, Prof Julian Marchesi; gut physiologists, Dr Mark Scott and Dr Anthony Hobson; gastroenterologists, Prof Douglas Drossman, Dr Shameer Mehta, Dr Farooq Rahman and Prof. David Sanders; and immunologist Dr Jenna Macciochi; thank you for sharing your brains. I have learnt so much from all of you.

Niki Webster and Renee Martensen, thank you for your game-changing flavours. To my family, friends and social media followers for being my recipe testers, and to Jessica Rowan-Parry and Claire Hitchen for reviewing my words – I truly valued every piece of feedback.

To my chapter contributors, Kimberly Wilson, Richie Norton, Dr Haya Al Khatib, Lucy Allen and Ellie Bradshaw, your additions have been instrumental in achieving my vision for a holistic guide to the gut.

To Penguin Life, Emily, Richard, Nic & Lou, Emma, Libby and the shoot team, what a journey – thank you for going that extra mile. John Hamilton, thank you for sharing your brilliance with me, I am forever grateful. RIP.

And finally, to each and every one of you that has supported *The Gut Health Doctor* journey. Thank you for believing in my mission – you are my driving force.